Secrets of Slender

*Ignite Your Fat-Burning Furnace
and Enrich Your Quality of Life*

Secrets of Slender

*Ignite Your Fat-Burning Furnace
and Enrich Your Quality of Life*

By Dr. Bryan Craig

This book is dedicated to...

My parents, who have always been a source of inspiration, support, and encouragement. Thank you, mom and dad, for always providing such a wonderful environment for me to always strive, grow, and be the best I can be!

To my dear friend, Anita, for your unconditional friendship, support, and encouragement.

To my friend, Ed, who has been a source of learning, inspiration, and support in many areas of my life. Many thanks for your encouragement and support in writing this book.

To The People:
Wake up and reclaim your health, vigor, and natural shape. It's your birthright!

Table of Contents

Disclaimer

The information contained in this book is provided for your general information only. It is not intended to be medical advice nor to engage in the practice of medicine. Under no circumstance is any information or advice contained in this book a recommendation for a particular treatment for a specific individual, and in all cases, you should consult your physician before pursuing any course of treatment or treatment program.

Introduction

The life we are experiencing is a gift, and it is up to us to determine what direction we want to go in and what we want to create. Our body carries us through the experiences life has to offer; it is the very mechanism by which we perceive and experience everything. We should treat ourselves with the respect and care that we deserve. Our body is one of a kind.

"How am I going to live today in order to create the tomorrow I'm committed to?"

Tony Robbins

I have seen much misinformation and confusion about what it takes to become slender or look our best while at least maintaining, if not, enhancing our health. I decided to write this book to share what I have learned in the hopes that it will touch and impact the lives of many in an effective, inspiring, and positive way. This is the type of book I wish were available to me in the midst of my confusion. I want to help you solve the problem of stubborn weight. The weight is really a symptom, the end result of a process, not the problem itself. You will learn that what controls metabolism are our hormones. You are going to learn how to make these hormones work for you instead of against you. We have hormones that trigger fat loss and those that make fat. It's critical to know how to trigger these fat-burning hormones in order to get slender. It's equally important to not sabotage your fat burning by triggering the hormones that make fat.

How did I learn about wellness and becoming slender? Through much trial and error.

Ever since I was young, I had an attraction towards natural health and fitness, so becoming a doctor of natural methods to encourage wellness was appealing to me. Due to having terrible problems with my back and headaches at a young age, my parents took me to see a chiropractor. When he pointed out a cause and effect relationship between my muscles, nerves, and joints to the back pain and headaches I was suffering with, I was amazed and intrigued. Each time I went in for a visit, I was significantly improved and couldn't wait to experience more of the wellness that I knew was inside of me. So when it was time to choose my profession, becoming a chiropractor seemed to be a perfect fit. Throughout my life, I always stayed in good shape and seemed to be healthy. I exercised regularly and paid attention to what I thought was proper nutrition.

It seemed that things started to change in my forties. I was perplexed. The diet and exercise methods that previously helped me stay in shape didn't seem to have the same effect any longer. I noticed a change in my energy levels, and I seemed to grow a belly. My routine hadn't changed, but my body did. Perhaps I wasn't doing everything I could for my shape and health to stay at its peak.

I started concentrating on my diet and changed my workouts, but my exercise time was becoming a burden. I still had some belly fat and my diet was not satisfying.

I decided that I needed to take a different approach and started to read different diet books, and, very quickly, I became very confused. It seemed that, outside of the basic advice to eat a healthy diet and exercise, there were many unanswered questions.

"Were carbohydrates good or bad?"

"Why do some runners die of heart disease?"

"Why do certain diets work for some people yet not for others?"

"Why did something that had worked for me for years all of a sudden seem to stop working?"

I needed to dig deeper so I returned to my basic human physiology books and examined what happens to the body on a cellular level when we eat and exercise.

A distinguishing factor was to apply the Pareto Principle, a simple formula used in business and in marketing that says *twenty percent of the work yields eighty percent of the results.*

I discovered common denominators such as low and no carb diets had the fastest weight loss. After my research, it became obvious how each diet and exercise program affected the body.

Now, I understood how low carb diets encouraged weight loss until you were left with those last few stubborn pounds. By applying the Pareto Principle, I learned I could limit carbs to twenty percent of the time when they were beneficial and lose that stubborn weight I wanted, without being tired or hungry. The reasons some diets worked and others didn't were not contradictory any longer; they became clear to me.

Through this book you will have the tools and understanding to make a plan so that you can get slender, healthy, fit, and look good—one that requires minimal exercise time and only a few simple eating principles. Being healthy and looking good doesn't require a lot of hard work, dedication, or giving up your favorite things. It only requires having the right information so you can make the best choices.

Until now, finding the right information was often harder than actually implementing it.

As you read this book, there probably will be some surprises. My principles might seem different than those you have heard before, but as I reveal the science behind them, they will start to make sense and you will wonder why it took so long for someone to reveal them in such a comprehensible and practical manner.

The truths and methods in this book can be followed for a lifetime. *This is not a crash diet or exercise routine, but a lifestyle that can and will give you the results you have been looking for!*

The basic concepts are simple and easy to learn. My approach shows you how to choose optimal foods and limit less than optimal foods to twenty percent of the time and when the best times are to indulge, should you so desire. The most basic idea is to let your body automatically manage its own blood sugar instead of you deliberately trying to manage your blood sugar with food intake. This will free you up from having to manage your weight, as most systems promote. These methods will also show you that you don't need to lose weight in order to become healthy; rather, as you do what is necessary to become healthier, your body will automatically drop the excessive weight!

With the news full of stories about the obesity epidemic, lost productivity due to health issues, and the economic burden of healthcare costs (which are actually sick care costs), not to mention the actual pain and suffering caused by health issues, it should seem obvious that being healthy should be a priority. The problem seems to be that most people don't have the information or the resources to make the correct choices that lead to better lifestyle.

If you have tried diet after diet and spent hours in the gym but never really solved your weight and health issues, or it was just too much work, then this book is for you. If you want to look vibrant and enrich your wellness, then this is the book for you. If you just want to make a few changes to help you look better, then this is the book for you. Even if you just want to know more about how to become slender and feel great but aren't ready to make any changes, then this is the book for you. The plan will be to keep it as simple and easy as possible.

Once I implemented the methods in this book into my lifestyle, I quickly reached my goals and found it very easy to maintain. Patients and friends started asking me to explain all of my "secrets" to them. They were intrigued and asked me if I had written these concepts and methods down. This was the impetus for me to write this book and to make sure it didn't stay a secret any longer. When you get healthy, "looking good" will follow naturally.

Not only will I give you steps to follow, I will give you examples along the way and tell you my choices for my own plan. I will teach you how to make your own plan, one that will work for you and that you will be able to easily stick to! Don't worry if you don't understand something; I've got your back. Just visit my website at www.secretsofslender.com and ask me any questions or discuss the principles in the book with others.

The principles in this book will help you enjoy these benefits:

Get leaner by burning fat

Enjoy better fitting clothes

Impact & balance hormonal levels

No need to count calories

Less hunger & more energy during the day

Look younger & more vibrant

Feel satisfied at the end of the day

Sharper thinking & deeper sleeping

Enrich your quality of life

Diet

In my application of the Pareto Principle, diet is 80 percent of your approach. Making some basic dietary changes will have the biggest impact and effect on your looks, weight, and health. But it doesn't have to be drastic or a sacrifice.

Some of my patients are always worried that they will have to give up everything they like or eat like a rabbit.

People want to feel better about the choices they make and that's important. Whether good or bad, you have to make some room in your eating plan for things you really want.

But one thing we all want is more time. This leads to a very important point: *All* foods promote aging. Of course, we still need to eat since foods provide energy and nutrients, but the body has a limited amount of cellular cycles to process the food. Every time you eat, you contribute to the aging process by using those cycles, so, from this perspective, no single food item is necessarily "healthy," but there are healthier food choices.

We need to evaluate which of the available foods are the best choices, how much to eat, and when to eat. The latter, *when to eat*, seems to be the most neglected and misunderstood aspect to eating, yet it is one of the most important.

In order to burn fat, our liver must be healthy. Why? All hormones that burn fat create their effects *through the liver*, which is why it's so important that this organ has proper health and function. It's virtually impossible to burn fat when the liver is not in good condition. If you ever want to spot a person whose liver isn't functioning very well, here are some key indicators: potbelly, brown spots on the back of the hands, red dots on different areas of the body, bad breath, low energy upon waking, yellowish tint in the whites of the eyes, and bad joints.

As you continue to get your liver in a healthier state, it's important to be aware of what can block your glands from functionally properly. What you should avoid: large amounts of alcohol; coffee and black tea; artificial fats; hydrogenated fats; margarine; deep fried fats; conventional vegetables and fruits (sprayed with many chemicals); (hormone-laden) eggs and meats or meats with nitrates; and pasteurized milk and chips. There are many substitutes you can enjoy such as green and/or herbal teas; real butter; coconut butter; flax, olive, coconut, and walnut oils; organic vegetables and fruits; fertile, cage free eggs; free range, organic meats; wild caught fish; and clean water.

Instinctual Eating

Our ancient ancestors lived and ate by instinct. Our bodies directed how we ate. It is my strong belief that as humans evolved over millennia we trained ourselves to change these natural instincts.

We know from historical records that many of our ancestors, including the Greeks and Romans, ate very little during the day while they hunted, marched, and trained, yet they had plenty of energy and strength. At night, they would set up camp and feast on the catch of the day.

Burning fat during the day gave them a strong, steady supply of energy. Occasionally getting hungry during the day probably gave them an edge without being a distraction. If mild or moderate hunger entered the mind, they would "scavenge" by eating berries along the way or some dried meat that they carried with them.

If the hunger did become stronger, it could be dismissed with the comforting knowledge that in the evening they would be enjoying a full belly. I have done this myself, and it worked for me too.

You can use this type of eating schedule to your advantage and benefit from a steady level of energy throughout the day. You can also use it to schedule favorite foods that are just for enjoyment as opposed to health.

Calorie Restriction

As mentioned earlier, every time you eat, you contribute to the aging process, so consuming as close to the minimum amount of calories that you actually need is optimal. Too few calories, as endorsed by certain crash diets, and you risk being malnourished, slowing your metabolism, and a breaking down tissues and muscle. Too many calories and you risk speeding up the aging process and storing fat.

There is a very helpful yet complex formula to determine how many calories you need. First, calculate your BMR or basal metabolic rate, and then multiply in factors such as your sex, age, height, and weight. Multiply that by your activity level and you have your calorie needs. Fortunately, you won't need to figure that out as long as you follow my principles, nor will *you need to worry about counting calories*. Just like riding a bike, you'll instinctively know when you've eaten enough as your system comes back into balance.

Poor, Adequate, and Optimal Nutrition

The benefit-to-aging ratio of each food determines whether it is a poor, adequate, or optimal choice. Choosing foods that provide optimal nutrition will provide the best health and slow aging. Choosing foods that are poor will not provide enough nourishment and force you to eat more to make up the difference. I've included a handy reference at the end of the book that lists which foods fall into each category.

Food Timing

Your body needs different types of energy and nutrients at different times. An important concept that is often forgotten is that the food you eat now is mostly for energy you will need later. Your body needs to process and store nutrients before it can use them. Timing your food consumption with these natural cycles can have a huge impact on your health, weight, strength, energy levels, longevity, and hunger cycles. Before you can start planning your food timing you'll need to understand the different types of foods and how they provide energy.

The main concept of food timing comes down to under-eating and over-eating cycles. As we learn about the different types of foods, I will refer to these cycles. Once we have reviewed all the food types, we will put it all together and learn about the cycles.

Q. Is it true that breakfast is the most important meal of the day?

A. In my opinion it is the least important meal of the day. Unless you are under nourished, the body should have plenty of stored energy and nutrients. That doesn't mean you need to skip it, you just need to eat appropriately so that your fat burning cycle will not be interfered with.

Food for Energy

There are two main types of fuel that your body uses for energy: Glucose (sugar) and fatty acids. The body uses these fuels to create adenosine triphosphate (ATP), which is the energy source of the body. Later in the book, I will explain the role of ATP in more detail.

Glucose comes from carbohydrates that are sugar or that break down into sugar, such as bread, pasta, rice, and cake. Glucose is stored in the liver as glycogen and can be released as needed to maintain blood sugar levels. Muscles have their own private stores of glycogen to use as energy when needed. Fatty acids generally come from animal products and from fat already stored in your body. A third type of less important fuel that the body uses is amino acids. Amino acids come from the breakdown of muscles and other tissue during times of starvation or over activity.

Glucose is very easy for the body to use as energy. Excess glucose is like afterburners on a fighter jet or nitrous oxide on a funny car. It provides a lot of energy, very quickly and for short periods of time. But, just like a jet can't run on afterburners for more than a short time, neither can our bodies. The body keeps five to ten grams of glucose in the blood to use when needed.

Fatty acids provide a steady, slow burning energy that lasts much longer. Ideally, your body uses fatty acids as its main source of energy. When the blood glucose levels are over about ten grams, the body stops burning fat and works to store the excess glucose, first as glycogen in the muscles and liver, then as fat.

When we are young, our bodies can easily revert from processing glucose to burning fat again. But, as we age, the body gets accustomed to the constant supply of excess sugar, and it will have a harder time using fat as an energy source.

Many people develop such difficulty in burning fat that they depend on a constant supply of dietary sugar as their main source of energy. Also, many times these people have tendencies towards hypoglycemia. They will often complain about low blood sugar and will find the need to eat constantly. The problem with sugar is that the body constantly strives to lower your blood sugar levels to less than ten grams. In other words, instead of your body regulating your blood sugar by raising it as needed, your eating habits have been raising your blood sugar, and now your body has adapted to that. In this state, the body never gets the chance to burn stored fat.

> *"Why is it so important for the body to lower blood sugar?" It is a paradox that some things the body needs are also toxic to it, even in limited excess. For example, mixed air divers are constantly worried about oxygen toxicity because too much oxygen is a toxin. Too much sugar is also a toxin; that's why the body is constantly trying to lower your blood sugar after eating. Excess glucose binds to proteins affecting their function. Just ask any diabetic about the effects of excess sugar on their kidneys, eyes, and general health and you will think twice about using sugar as your main source of fuel.*

Insulin and Glucagon

The body uses insulin and glucagon to regulate metabolism. They are the main hormones created in the pancreas.

The body releases insulin to lower blood sugar as a safety measure. When you're hungry and you eat something that elevates your blood sugar, there is now too much toxic sugar in your blood, so your body releases insulin to lower those levels. It only takes about ten grams of sugar to raise your blood sugar to the point where a significant amount of insulin will be released. A can of soda, a candy bar, or two slices of bread will all raise your blood sugar enough to release insulin. Later in the book you will learn a simple guideline to determine how much a food with affect your blood sugar.

With excess insulin, your blood sugar drops. Unless your body is adept at turning back to burning fat, you become tired and hungry, so you eat some more food that elevates your blood sugar and your body releases more insulin. And this cycle goes on and on. Instead of allowing your body to regulate blood sugar normally, you are forcing your body to constantly respond to changes in blood sugar.

In order to lower your blood sugar, insulin converts sugar to fat in the blood, in the form of cholesterol and triglycerides. You might think that the body uses that fat for energy, but it can't. It uses those saturated fats in the liver for hormone production or stores it for a "rainy day." But if you are regularly eating foods that elevate blood sugar, there is never a "rainy day," and your body "forgets" how to use the fat for energy. So you end up storing a lot of fat and never using it.

Insulin is not very good at regulating blood sugar.
But it is very good at lowering blood sugar and
storing sugar as saturated fat.

A sugary diet will lead to a lot of insulin being produced to lower blood sugar. Eventually, the cells become resistant to the effects of insulin, which leads to a very common illness called insulin-resistant diabetes. The body produces a lot of insulin to regulate blood sugar, but it doesn't lower blood sugar levels.

What many people don't know is that lowering blood sugar is only a very small part of what insulin does. In fact, insulin can have an effect on virtually all body functions, and the body is constantly releasing a small amount of insulin to handle these. If the body does not have enough insulin, such as in periods of starvation, then the body will release cortisol to break down tissue for fuel. Cortisol causes depression and fatigue as your body tries to slow your metabolism and conserve energy; it also causes fat storage.

Cells in the human body split into new cells in order to replace dying or dead cells. That is the basic aging process. Over time, the cells have split so many times that they don't function as well as they once did. Insulin is what the body uses to split those cells. Insulin is actually short for Insulin Growth Factor (IGF). If your body is constantly producing excess insulin to lower your blood sugar, then all of that extra insulin will be around to age your cells faster. Eating a diet that releases a lot of insulin will cause your body to age faster.

Heart disease and cardiovascular disease are major health problems in this country, and doctors will tell you that high cholesterol and triglycerides are the cause. We just learned that blood cholesterol and triglycerides come from insulin transporting the sugar through the blood to be stored, so eating a diet that releases a lot of insulin will cause cardiovascular problems.

When your body is exposed to any toxins, it will store them in saturated fat and may mutate the cells to contain the toxins. Those mutated cells are called cancer cells. Humans have always had cancer cells, and their presence in the body is normal. What isn't normal is for them to grow. Some types of cancers like prostate, breast, and colorectal are particularly addicted to sugar and these cancer cells have a huge demand for insulin. If your body is constantly releasing extra insulin, it will be around to feed those cancer cells. In other words, eating a diet that releases a lot of insulin will increase your production of certain cancer cells.

Glucagon is the hormone that the body uses to burn fat and raise blood sugar. Glucagon is very good at regulating blood sugar. So, if your body is busy releasing excess insulin, glucagon (the fat burning hormone) will not get released. If you want your body to burn fat, you need it to be able to *turn glucagon back on* quickly.

The best way to get your body to release glucagon is to manage your carbohydrate consumption.

Q. If I am diabetic, can I follow these principles?

A. Since the focus of diabetic treatment is to regulate blood sugar and the principles in this book are designed to do just that, it follows that this would be a great lifestyle for a diabetic. However, the best plan for a diabetic would be the elimination of all sugar and non-fiber carbohydrates.

Leptin, Serotonin, and Cholecystokinin

Leptin is the hormone that the body releases when you are burning fat. It helps control hunger, appetite, and metabolism. If you don't eat enough calories, your body will not release enough leptin and you will be hungry. If an individual is overweight, the cells eventually become *resistant* to leptin, and even though you release it, it doesn't register and therefore doesn't suppress your hunger. Once your body resumes using fat for energy, your leptin levels will be more stable and you won't be as hungry. Consuming appetite suppressants do not deal with this problem at the root cause nor can they ever be a true source of correction for the body's hormone imbalance. The methods I'm teaching you will activate your own natural appetite suppressants without any negative side effects!

Serotonin is a mood-enhancing hormone. When serotonin levels are high, you are in a good mood. When they are low, you are in a bad mood. Certain foods help serotonin levels, such as pineapples, walnuts, bananas, kiwis, plums, and tomatoes. Unfortunately, non-fiber carbohydrates have a huge effect on serotonin levels, and that's why we tend to crave them and call them "comfort foods." Knowing how to consume these types of foods is critical for your overall success.

Cholecystokinin is released from the intestines during the digestion of fat and protein. It stimulates the release of digestive enzymes and bile. It also acts as a hunger suppressant. If you try to limit your calories excessively, your body will not release cholecystokinin and you will be hungry, locked into this vicious cycle.

Sleep is also an important part of leptin and serotonin production, and that's just another reason why you need a good night's sleep.

Cortisol and Ketones

Although they have several functions in the body, our main concern is that the body releases cortisol and ketones when it needs to conserve calories and energy. The body needs to release them when you consume too few calories over a period of time. They have a catabolic (breaking down) effect on the body and ultimately decrease metabolism, which is why crash diets are dangerous to your health and ineffective at solving weight issues. If you drastically cut your calories for too long a period, your body goes into survival mode. Since it thinks it has to conserve energy, it will do everything it can to store energy, not burn it. This is why you cannot lose fat in this manner and expect it to stay off. Most diet approaches don't address how you will take care of yourself long term; they only address immediate results. You cannot assume that internal balance and health is present just because you may have reduced weight from a crash type of diet. It's been shown that the body will pack on harder fat once a crash diet cycle is completed in defense of future starvation. This is just the opposite of what people are looking for!

Estrogen and Testosterone

Estrogen has very important functions in the body, but like oxygen, sugar, and insulin, even a small excess of estrogen can have a very harmful effect. Estrogen has been linked to many diseases, cancers, infertility, and obesity. Certain foods and chemicals will stimulate the production of estrogen in the body.

Our modern world of plastics, chemicals, and radiation constantly acts to increase the production of estrogen. Processing of our foods with hormones, chemicals, and radiation, using chemical cleaners, and radiation exposure from natural and man-made sources have made it impossible to avoid exposure completely. There are some steps that you can take to limit your exposure. Since plastic is the biggest source of chemicals that stimulate the release of estrogen, store your food in non-plastic containers. Try to purchase fruits, vegetables, and animal products that are not sold in plastic, nor are mass-produced, fed hormones, antibiotics, or irradiated.

Many skin creams, sunscreen, and hair products are loaded with chemicals such as p-nonylphenol. Using these products is like rubbing liquid plastic on your skin.

Q. I heard that sunscreen causes cancer, is that true?

A. Sunlight in moderation is an important part of a healthy lifestyle. How much is moderation? If your skin turns lightly tan, that is okay. If it turns red, that's too much. The best way to avoid too much exposure is to limit exposure to the sun and wear clothing that blocks the sun. Slobbering chemicals all over your skin that stimulate estrogen production and can react with the sunlight to cause free radicals is not my idea of a safety measure, whether or not they protect from or cause skin cancer. If you need to use them, use them sparingly and make sure that they protect across the full spectrum.

Some foods also have an estrogen stimulation effect. The most common are soy, hops, alcohol, and vegetable oils like soy, canola, safflower, and corn.

> *Beer is one of the most popular beverages that contain both hops and alcohol. I'm sure you have seen many beer bellies. I'm not saying you have to give up beer, but if you want to be slender and healthier, beer is not the best choice. If you are a real beer drinker, you probably know that the pale beers are high in hops and dark beers are high in barley. If you do choose to drink beer, you can make a better choice by choosing a darker beer. Unfortunately, beer ranks high on the estrogenic scale.*

Testosterone also has many important functions in the body. Unfortunately, as we age, testosterone production declines. A diet high in good fat and protein and low in non-fiber carbohydrates (more about these later), coupled with proper exercise and sleep, will help keep testosterone production near peak levels and reduce the effects of the aging process. (Women, tell your men about this!)

Proteins

Amino acids are the building blocks of protein, and although proteins can provide fuel, they are a last resort fuel source for the body. The main benefit of proteins is that they provide the building blocks for repairing the body.

Protein is vital. Vegetables provide a small amount of protein, beans provide a little more, and raw seeds and nuts are a very good source.

While peanuts are often confused as a nut, they are actually a fruit, part of the legume family with beans and not as high in protein as true nuts.

The primary source of protein is from eating fish and meat, including their milk and eggs. These provide the highest amount of protein per calorie. Getting enough protein may be a challenge for vegans and some vegetarians, but this can be compensated for by eating nuts, beans, and quality protein supplements.

Bee pollen, one of my favorites, is an all-natural super vitamin. It contains every nutrient needed by humans. It also has one of the highest percentages of protein per gram from any food source. It comes in granular form and can be purchased from your local honey farmer. It's always best to consume locally grown bee pollen respective to where you live.

There is a problem with eating meat, and that is saturated fat, not to mention the hormones and other chemicals in conventional meats. Animals in the wild consume very little carbs or sugar, but animals raised for food are fed huge amounts of *grain*, which elevates their blood sugar and releases a lot of insulin. All of that extra sugar is stored as saturated fat. That's why saturated fat tastes good: it is actually processed and concentrated sugar. That's also why it is bad for you. Grass-fed animals don't store much saturated fat and are a better source of healthy protein. It's always better to choose grass-fed beef when making your purchase. True, it costs more, however, that's a decision you must make about what your priorities are.

Because proteins are easily absorbed by your body, they don't really interfere with fats or carbohydrates and can be eaten at any time. Moreover, they are very important when the body needs a supply of building blocks, such as during sleep, illness, and after exercising.

Fats

Fats are the *best* energy source for the body, but not all fats are created equal.

Good sources of fat are fatty fish, such as salmon and Chilean Sea Bass, avocadoes, coconuts, olives, seeds, nuts, and olive oil. The best source of fat is the fat already stored in your body!

Bad sources of fats include all fried foods, vegetable oils, and grain-fed animal products.

The best part about fats is that you won't intentionally need to include them into your meal plans. When you make healthier food choices, the right amount of good fats will automatically be in your diet.

Carbohydrates

Carbohydrates are often categorized as simple or complex. Simple carbs are sugars: candy, cakes, cookies, syrup, and sodas. Complex carbs, also referred to as starch, are foods that will be broken down into sugars, such as bread, pasta, rice, and most fruits and vegetables. Ultimately, sugar carbs and starch carbs are the same thing because they both end up as sugar in the blood. I prefer instead to categorize them as fiber and non-fiber carbohydrates.

Fiber carbs are those that don't break down into sugar, like the fiber found in vegetables.

Non-fiber carbs (Sugar/Starch/Complex) are the "bad" carbs that do break down into sugar, such as potatoes, flour, corn, rice, pasta, breads, cake, and candy.

> *I want to mention that corn is **not** a vegetable. Corn is a grain and would fall under the non-fiber carb category. Unfortunately, our society treats corn as a vegetable, and because it is cheap to produce, it is overly abundant in our diet.*

Fiber carbs are always the best choice. They can be eaten any time during the day, and they don't significantly affect your blood sugar or insulin levels.

Non-fiber, starch, complex, and sugar carbs all affect your blood sugar and will cause insulin to be released. The carbohydrate choices that you make will have the biggest impact on your health. Not just in what you eat, but *when* you eat them because there are times, such as after exercise, when the body needs to raise your blood sugar quickly.

Brown rice, yams, and dark breads like pumpernickel, German dark wheat, and the Ezekiel brand, commonly found in the freezer at health food stores, are some of the better choices for starchy carbohydrates. They have a higher quantity of fiber and less overall sugar.

There are no good choices for sugar carbs! Sugar carbs are the *empty calories* so often talked about, and they have little place in a healthy diet. If you want to enjoy them, you'll have to be careful about how often and when you eat them. But those starchy and sugary carbs sure are delicious, comfort foods. Surely there must be a time and place for them. While there is never a perfect time for them, there are times when starch carbohydrates can actually be used to your advantage.

For example, immediately after a workout your body is working to *release* blood sugar. Glucagon is converting stored fat into glucose, and insulin is working to replenish the depleted glycogen stores. Twenty to thirty grams of starchy carbohydrates shortly after a workout will help replenish your depleted muscle glycogen stores. *This is the best time to schedule some starch carbohydrates*. The best choice would be a high-fiber, low-sugar bread, but you could also use this time to schedule a dessert or treat.

As discussed earlier, when you eat non-fiber starch carbs, you spike your blood sugar and provide a boost of energy. In response, your body releases insulin, which drops your blood sugar and tends to make you tired and hungry. During the day, being tired and hungry is probably not ideal, but this is what happens when we eat a big breakfast or lunch. However, shortly after dinner you will have a full belly and are getting ready to go to sleep. Eating some starch carbs at dinner won't stimulate your appetite if you're sleeping, and this meal will help you get to sleep. This would be the *next best time* to eat non-fiber, starch carbs.

Even better would be the *evening before* a calorie-burning activity, such as a bike ride or run. This insures that your muscle's glycogen stores are full and that stored energy will be available to burn during the activity. When you eat, the immediate energy from the food is minimal, and most of the energy is meant to be stored for future use.

> *The best time to eat starch carbs is shortly after a workout. There is a window of thirty to sixty minutes to eat up to thirty grams of non-fiber carbs following a workout.*

If you have a lot of fat to lose, or are having trouble with those last few pounds, the fastest and healthiest way to lose it is to completely avoid non-fiber, complex, and sugar carbohydrates until you reach your goal. The only exception to this is after working out. You should always eat some starch carbs and protein after working out.

Glycemic Index and Load

As we discussed earlier, the body keeps five to ten grams of glucose in the blood for normal use. When it gets higher than that, extra insulin is released. The glycemic index and load refer to how much a certain food will raise your blood sugar and for how long. Candy, which is almost pure sugar, will raise the blood sugar quickly, but only for a short time. Yams will raise the blood sugar much less, but for much longer.

This is important because fifteen grams of sugar, such as that found in a candy bar, will raise your blood sugar and definitely cause the release of extra insulin. The body will then quickly lower the blood sugar and start storing it. This makes you tired and hungry again.

Fifteen grams of starch carbs, such as a sweet potato, will enter the blood stream more slowly and may not raise the blood sugar high enough at any time to release extra insulin.

However, a hundred grams of a starch carb, such as pasta, will spike your insulin over a long period of time. This will cause you to store most of the food for future use, but it is less likely to make you tired or hungry.

A Quick Reference Insulin Index:
I have a handy rule of thumb to determine the
likelihood of releasing extra insulin. I take the total
grams of carbohydrates on the food label, add the
sugar grams, and minus the fiber grams. I call the
result the insulin index. If it is from zero to ten, then
it is unlikely that extra insulin will be released. If it
is between ten and twenty, then it is possible. If it is
between twenty and thirty, then it is probable. If it is
over thirty, then insulin will definitely be released.
Twenty is the magic number to remember, so try
and keep the insulin index under twenty during any
one-hour period

Fiber

Fiber is a carbohydrate that the body *does not digest,* so it does not break down into sugar and does not affect insulin levels. There are two types of fiber: soluble and non-soluble.

Soluble fiber comes mostly from vegetables and fruits. It dissolves in water and helps to soften the stool.

Non-soluble fiber comes mostly from seeds, nuts, grains, and vegetables. It does not dissolve in water and helps form the stool and clean the intestines.

When you look at the nutrition label, the amount of fiber will be listed under carbohydrates. The higher the fiber content, the better!

Q. If I eat more whole grains, which contain heart-healthy fiber as well as vitamins and minerals, will it help me stay full between meals?

A. For about an hour. The problem with all of that grain is that even though it has fiber, it still has non-fiber carbs. It is likely to spike your blood sugar, and your body will respond by releasing insulin, which will then lower your blood sugar and make you hungry again. Whole grains are better choices for your non-fiber starch carbs, but should only be eaten during the carb friendly times.

Omega-6 and Omega-3

There are two fats that your body cannot make and are classified as essential: the Omega-3 and Omega-6 fatty acids. They are both important, and each has a very different effect on the body.

Omega-6 fatty acids, such as those found in processed foods like potato chips, stimulate the release of cytokines, which have an inflammatory effect on the body. In excess, Omega-6 fatty acids can be toxic and produce many problematic issues in the body, even bad skin! If you see someone who has acne, that is a sign that they might very well have too much Omega-6 fatty acids causing an inflammatory response; it can also indicate a sluggish liver. While inflammation is part of the early healing process, too much inflammation will lead to arthritis, autoimmune diseases, pain, and many other problems. They also stimulate the production of estrogen.

Omega-3 fatty acids, such as those found in salmon and olive oil, have an anti-inflammatory effect on the body. Another lesser-known source of Omega-3 is grass or pasture fed beef and game. They help the body with the later stages of healing and inhibit the release of estrogen.

The typical American diet is high in Omega-6 fatty acids and low in Omega-3 fatty acids. Concentrating on increasing Omega-3 intake and using Omega-3 supplements is good way to make up for the shortage of Omega-3 fatty acids and is often suggested by many experts. However, decreasing the intake of Omega-6 is the other half of the equation. The biggest sources of Omega-6 in your diet are starch carbs, vegetable oils, and processed foods such as cookies and chips—you know, the stuff that is available from supermarkets to gas stations! These foods tend to have long shelf lives and should be another indication that it is not designed as a good choice for human consumption.

Breakfast, Lunch, and Dinner

A typical *poor* diet might look something like this:

Breakfast:

Buttered roll with bacon and fruit juice. Other typical breakfast foods include bagels, cereals, Danishes, pastries, waffles, and pancakes and syrup.

Lunch:

Sandwich of processed meat, bag of chips, soda or beer.

Dinner:

Pizza and beer. Spaghetti and meatballs. Steak (hormone laden) and potatoes.

This provides a steady supply of sugar all day that will cause the body to release insulin and store fat. Over time, insulin resistance is likely to develop.

> *Your body burns fat to raise your blood sugar. If your body is constantly working to lower your blood sugar, it never has any reason to burn fat. This is how that stubborn, hard fat forms and the reason why it doesn't easily leave the body!*

Many people think that they can't change their diet because they will miss eating certain foods or crave them. The truth is that taste is acquired, especially sweetness, and it can be changed, perhaps more easily than you think. If you eat something that you don't care for, over time, you can develop a taste for it. Even if you can't give up particular foods, knowing the best times to eat them can still make a big impact.

For example, years ago I enjoyed my coffee light, with sugar. Black coffee tasted horrible to me. Over time, I slowly cut back on the sugar, until I no longer added it, and then I cut back on the milk until I no longer added that. Eventually, I started drinking my coffee black, and now I prefer it that way.

Some people fear that they will be hungry all the time. When your blood sugar is fluctuating because you are using food intake to regulate it, your leptin and serotonin levels will cause you to crave food, especially starchy carbohydrates. But if your blood sugar is stable and you are eating enough calories, your leptin and serotonin levels are more stable, you won't be hungry, and your body won't crave food. You see, eating is a hormonal event.

Live Food vs. Dead Food

Live foods are simply foods that were alive and are usually eaten raw, such as vegetables or berries. They can be cooked, but usually only minimally, such as grilled fish or vegetables.

Foods that are processed are dead foods. Seeds are live foods, but seeds ground up into flour and baked into bread are dead foods. When you go to the supermarket, most of the food around the perimeter is live food, and the food in the aisles is dead food.

During your under-eating cycle, try to eat only live foods and snacks.

During your over-eating phase, try to eat live foods first, and then you can finish with dead foods, if you wish.

There is a detailed list of foods later in the book to help you choose.

Fruit

Fruit is a complex food. On the one hand, they are live and also great sources of fiber, nutrients, and antioxidants. On the other hand, they can affect blood sugar.

> *During the day it is best to eat only high-nutrient, high-fiber, low-sugar fruits such as berries or apples. When you do eat fruits, limit them to one piece or a half-cup serving.*

In the evening, during your over-eating phase, you can enjoy a higher-sugar fruit, but again, limit the serving to one or two pieces or a cup. Over the course of the day, a total of three pieces of fruit is acceptable. Choose organic whenever possible to avoid all of the commercial sprays.

Because of their higher concentration of sugar, dried fruits should be avoided or strictly limited.

Vegetables

I have nothing bad to say about vegetables. Fresh or salt-free frozen vegetables are optimal food choices and can be eaten anytime and in any amount. I don't think you need to worry about eating too many vegetables. Organic is a superior choice than conventionally grown due to all of the sprays, pesticides, etc. We don't benefit by consuming all of those chemicals and are likely to store them in our tissues and raise estrogen levels. I recommend consuming sprouted vegetables, such as broccoli and/or alfalfa sprouts. Sprouts are one of the most nutrient packed foods because they are loaded with enzymes and anticancer properties. Sprouts have been found to contain up to one hundred times the anticancer properties than that of its mature form, which is the standard broccoli heads you see in the market. Sprouts are quicker and easier to eat while getting more nutrition. There are times people have a difficult time digesting certain vegetables and beans and bloating can occur. You can supplement your diet with high quality digestive enzymes.

Dairy

The nice thing about most cheeses is that they don't significantly affect your blood sugar, so, in limited quantities, they can be part of a healthy diet. Because it is processed, cheese is technically a dead food, but the way it is made allows it to be eaten during the live food phase in small quantities. Cheddar is probably one of the best choices; American cheese is the worst, as it is very heavily processed. Adding two ounces of cheese to your daily plan is fine. While plain yogurt could be an acceptable choice, unfortunately, name brand flavored yogurts are loaded with sugar, so be careful and read the label. Sour cream or cream cheese can be another acceptable choice.

Fermented and Pickled Foods

Although fermented foods such as cheese and pickles are processed, fermenting can add benefits to food. Certain anti-oxidants and friendly bacteria are only found in naturally fermented foods. Adding certain live foods that have been fermented into your diet—see examples below— can be a good choice. I've listed more of these in the detailed food list later in the book.

Here are some examples of good fermented foods:

- Vegetables into pickles, natural sauerkraut.
- Dairy into cheese, yogurt.

Here are some examples of other fermented foods:

- Beans into miso, tofu, soy sauce.
- Grains into beer, bread, rice wine, whisky.
- Fruits into wine, vinegar, brandy.
- Honey into mead.

A Note about Water

Keeping our hydration level is important. I have noticed that there has been a big push for everyone to consume more and more water. Drinking to attempt to satisfy hunger will not work for more than five minutes or so. Drinking too much water can actually make you feel bloated and give the appearance of small rings around the lower legs and ankles, most noticeable at night. Drinking too much water can also produce dehydration, just the opposite effect, by flushing out minerals which are responsible for holding the water in our system. So there is no need to force yourself to drink water, just pay attention to your body and drink when thirsty. Eating nutrient dense foods will help to maintain hydration levels.

In order to promote improved liver function, I recommend drinking, on an empty stomach 1-2x per day, a mixture of 6-8 oz. of water with 2 oz. of unsweetened non-concentrate cranberry juice (this is the bitter tasting cranberry juice, do not consumed the sweetened type). In addition, add 1 oz. of raw, unfiltered apple cider vinegar and squeeze lemon into the mix. This will add some great potassium into your system and promote flushing out of waste products while adding friendly bacteria to your system.

When Starting Your Plan, Timing Is Critical

Natural Cycles of Over-Eating and Under-Eating

Now that we know how the body uses certain types of foods, we can start our plan. The over-eating phase should be twenty percent of our day, but we should consume eighty percent of our calories in that time period. First, we need to schedule an over-eating time; this is where the Calorie Shifting Method comes in. For most people, between 6:00 pm and 10:00 pm is the optimal time. During that period you may eat as much live food, protein, and vegetables as you desire. Once you are finished, you can eat some starchy carbs, then dessert. Ideally, you would limit the starch carbs to one cup and have only a small portion of dessert. A common approach is to be strict during the week and take some liberties on the weekend, but you can, of course, customize your approach to your lifestyle. The order in which you eat your food is not critical, but because live foods move through your digestive system faster, it is better for your digestion to consume them first. Also, if you fill up on the live foods, you are less likely to over eat the other foods.

> *During the under-eating phase, which is any time of day other than the over-eating phase, you want to limit yourself to live foods only. You should also limit the quantity, eating just enough to give your stomach a "feel" for what is to come later in the evening. During the day, I try to limit snacks to about one hundred calories, or meals to a fist-sized quantity per hour.*

Now, let's say that you have an event on Saturday; you'll be at a restaurant at noon and then eating all day. You're paying for a fancy meal, and you want to enjoy it. You can. Just make the day before or the day after an *all under-eating day*. During the under-eating days, eat only live foods (see the food list), avoid all non-fiber, starch carbs, and do not schedule an over-eating phase.

> *How can you tell when you've eaten enough during the over-eating phase? If you start to feel thirsty, you've eaten enough, and if you start to feel bloated, you've likely eaten too much.*

Over time, your *natural instinct* to know when you've eaten the right amount will come back and let you know when you are satisfied. Where did they go? Social conventions and modern lifestyle have trained you to ignore them, but they were always there because it's programmed within us. You can help yourself by taking smaller portions and resting between them. This will give you a chance to notice any changes, like thirst or bloating. We really do not require the volume of food to be consumed as most of our society tends to. By under-eating throughout the day and then shifting to your main meal for dinner, you will create a shift in your metabolism; this is the Calorie Shifting Method. It causes your body to start processing and utilizing nutrients, which will work for you instead of against you.

It might sound like the under-eating phase will be difficult, but the exact opposite is true. By eating foods that do not affect your blood sugar, your cravings will disappear. It might be strange the first few days, but after that it becomes quite natural.

Like many mammals, humans are naturally nocturnal (night) eaters. We are instinctively programmed to be active during the day, eat at night, then sleep. It is only because of the availability of food and our societal system that we eat all day. There is an actual disorder called Night Eating Syndrome, but I get the feeling that this might just be a label that describes people who are having trouble fighting their natural instincts.

Q. My family gets together every Sunday. We make a huge dinner with lots of great tasting non-fiber, starchy carbohydrates. How can I enjoy this yet not sabotage my results?

A. If at all possible, eat the live foods first and eat the non-fiber, starch carbs last. You will fill up on the healthier choices and eat less of the non-fiber, starch carbs. Depending upon the order the meal is served, that might not work. The next part of the solution is to plan Sunday as an over-eating day. To compensate, plan Saturday as an under-eating day and Monday as a high activity day.

Exercise

Much like food, everyday activity also contributes to the aging process. That doesn't mean you shouldn't exercise, but rather, that you should exercise effectively.

Proper exercise can and should build a strong heart and lungs, increase your metabolism, increase your strength, increase your energy, balance hormone levels, improve your overall health, and make you look healthier and younger. What follows is a plan to exercise effectively and safely.

High Intensity Interval Training (HIIT)

Our ancestors were hunters who were largely sedentary for many hours until they came across some prey, and then they would go into *quick action* to catch it. In these times, we behave in a similar way. We sit or stand all day and then need a burst of full energy to run up a flight of stairs, run after a taxi, or catch up with the kids. Rarely do we ever need the ability to run at a steady pace for mile after mile, except in an endurance sport. In fact, even most sports require only quick bursts of energy, such as tennis, baseball, golf, etc. Even sexual activities require only quick bursts of activity. Yet, most of our health-related exercise revolves around some type of repetitive, endurance activity.

So why do we do it? The first reason we give is to lose weight by burning calories. Well, at the gym, most people on the treadmill or stationary bike are actually burning only about three hundred calories an hour. It isn't hard to eat an extra three hundred calories, and the endurance training in itself tends to make you hungry. So, rather than losing weight, endurance training can lead to weight gain. It is a lot easier to just skip the three hundred calories than to run the hour, and a lot healthier too.

Controversial? Yes, but read on and you will understand more.

Another reason we say we work out is to raise metabolism or improve cardiovascular fitness. Wrong! The true measure of cardiovascular fitness is *recovery time*. If you and an elite sprinter both run fast for one minute, you will both increase your heart and respiration rates. The difference is the athlete's heart and respiratory rate will recover quicker. If you train for recovery time, you won't be winded for a long time after climbing a flight of stairs or running for a bus.

But, if all you do is walk or run or ride long distances at a steady pace, you never increase your metabolism, nor strengthen your heart, and you never improve recovery time. In fact, what you do is make your heart and lungs more efficient, and they actually get downsized.

> *More efficient means a slower metabolism and means you burn **less** calories. More efficient means smaller. Instead of building your heart and lungs, you are actually making them smaller and weaker over time.*

These types of activities are incorrectly called "cardio," when they are actually endurance type training. It is far better to exercise in *short bursts*, for example, sprinting.

Another reason we like to exercise is to strengthen joints and muscles. But repeating the same movements over and over puts wear and tear on your body, and your muscles adapt to those movements. That changes the muscles and joints, which start to function best only for that particular activity, instead of all activities.

Yet, if you have ever gone to the gym, you will see many overweight people running on treadmills, step machines, and stationary bikes for hours and hours. Many have been doing it for years and yet, they are still overweight. Endurance training does not increase your metabolism and does not burn enough calories to regulate your weight. So, exercising in this manner to control weight is really a poor choice.

Rather than exercising for long periods of time at a steady pace, I recommend exercising for less time with short bursts of high activity, followed by periods of recovery. This is called High Intensity Interval Training (HIIT), and it involves moving your body quickly to increase your heart rate. If done correctly, you can be finished in just ten minutes a day, three or four times per week. Even better, you won't need special equipment or a gym membership.

> *High Intensity Interval Training helps you build a strong heart, strong muscles, and stay lean. HIIT, and also resistance training, increases the thickness of the walls of the heart. The heart is a muscle and thicker walls mean more muscle. These beneficial changes can last for months even after training is stopped.*

> *While endurance training may increase the overall size of the heart, it does this by increasing the size of the left ventricle only, not the walls of the heart. The walls of the heart actually get smaller. When you stop endurance training, the left ventricle quickly returns to normal size.*

A High Intensity Interval Training (HIIT) session consists of a two-minute warm-up, followed by one to nine sets of intervals. Those sets can include any activity that you enjoy as long as it can be performed at an intensity that cannot be maintained for longer than one minute. They can be as simple as jumping rope or flipping tires. One of my favorites is to swim a lap/s HIIT style. It is low impact and really gets the heart and lungs engaged.

> *An interval set consists of a short burst of high activity followed by a period of recovery.*

The normal range of time for the burst of high activity is ten to thirty seconds. The period of recovery depends on your level of fitness and can range from thirty seconds to a few minutes.

ATP, the Energy Source of the Body

These high activity times aren't chosen randomly. ATP is the energy source of the body, and the body has different processes to use ATP. The amount of time that we can perform activities is limited by how long the cells can continue those processes.

Starting Your HIIT Program

The first step is to choose what exercises you will do during the high activity time.

When choosing exercises, the only criterion is that it has to be *challenging*. Be creative in your choices, and make them fun. You'll find that plyometric exercises such as squat thrust presses can be fun, challenging, and make your muscles powerful. There are many plyometric exercises to choose from.

Some of my favorites are:
- Band punches/presses
- Chin up/Pull ups
- Four point jumping jacks
- Frog jumps
- Kettle Bell swings
- Lateral jumps
- One legged jumps
- Push ups/clapping push ups

Once you've decided on your exercises, it is time to perform them.

I'm going to explain things as if you are an absolute beginner who has a very low level of cardiovascular fitness. If you are already exercising, you may be able to move through the steps more quickly. If you don't feel like you are ready for the next step, just repeat the current step or increase the recovery time accordingly.

The first goal is to get to three sets. Here are the steps to get there:

Let's say you've chosen to sprint. On day one, after your two-minute warm-up, which could be an easily paced jog, start sprinting *as fast as you can*. When you start to fade, feel winded, breath heavy, feel your pulse rate climb rapidly, or reach thirty seconds, STOP. Look at your time. In this example, we'll say you were able to run for ten seconds. That was your high activity time. Now, walk for at least a minute. This is your *recovery time*. You now have a starting point for your program. You can use the chart below to progress:

Week	High Activity Time in Seconds	Recovery Time in Seconds	Number of Sets
1	10	60	1
2	10	60	2
3	10	60	3
4	10	45	3
5	20	45	3
6	30	45	3
7	30	30	3

If you are unable to complete a set, increase your recovery time until your fitness improves. HIIT should be the basis for your healthy exercise plan, and, applying the Pareto principle, it should take about twenty percent of your exercise time but will account for eighty percent of the benefit. You should be doing your HIIT three or four times per week and allowing for a day of rest in between. If you aren't going to do any resistance training or endurance training as discussed in the next sections, you can perform HIIT every day, with just one day of rest per week.

Once you've reached the seventh week, you've reached your first goal. If you are a moderately active person and want to achieve a higher level of cardiovascular fitness, you can continue onto the next goal:

Week	High Activity Time in Seconds	Recovery Time in Seconds	Number of Sets
8, 9, 10	30	30	4
11, 12, 13	30	30	5
14	30	30	6

Once you are at this level, the cardiovascular gains have almost reached their peak, and there is no need for additional sets. If you are an athlete, you might want to perform up to nine sets to maximize the cardiovascular fitness, but after that, you are moving from high intensity interval training and into endurance training.

If you are serious about being healthy, we shouldn't
even have to discuss smoking. But, it is true that a
smoker who performs HIIT as described above will
most likely have better cardiovascular fitness than a
non-smoker who does not regularly perform HIIT.
That said, if you want to be healthy and look good,
give up smoking.

Q. I've chosen some HIIT exercises, but they don't get my heart rate up after several thirty-second intervals. What am I doing wrong?

A. Either the exercises aren't challenging enough or you aren't trying hard enough. You can try more challenging exercises, push yourself harder, or extend the high intensity interval time.

HIIT Exercises

Jumping jacks, jump rope, sprints, squat thrust presses, and pushups are the staple of body weight HIIT exercises. They can be done almost anywhere without special equipment. As you become more conditioned, you may want more challenging exercises or possibly are just bored with the basic exercises. Here are some examples of HIIT exercises, which can be referenced via the internet, Some require special equipment, some don't, but they are fun, challenging, and work the full body, including the core:

Alternating Thrusts:
1. Start in a pre-pushup position
2. Bring one knee forward and back (the knee should not touch the ground)
3. Bring the other knee forward and back (the knee should not touch the ground)
4. For a greater core workout, bring the knee toward the opposite elbow

One Leg Pushups:
1. Perform a normal pushup

   2. Try a variation of lifting a leg

   3. Try variations of hand positions, wide space, close space, further forward, further back

Clapping Pushups:

   1. Perform a normal pushup

   2. Push up quickly and try to clap your hands

Kettle Bell Swings:

   1. Start in a half squat position with the kettle bell between your legs.

   2. Push up quickly and swing the kettle bell out in front of you (be sure to keep your spine straight)

   3. Return to the starting position

Heavy Ropes:

   1. Stand with one rope in each hand

   2. Pull out all the slack from the rope

   3. Move forward until the rope is touching the ground one foot in front of your feet

Heavy ropes can be used in a variety of different ways.

   1. Alternate whipping each rope, creating waves

   2. Lift both ropes together and slam them down

   3. Alternate over hand or under grips

   4. Stand on one leg

   5. Make circles

   6. Squat or jump up and down while whipping the ropes

TRX:

TRX or similar strap systems you can perform rows, presses, planks, and many other exercises.

Sleds:

   1. Load an appropriate amount of weight on the sled (start with one quarter of your body weight)

2.   Hold the bar firmly. Try different grips, high and low

3.   Sprint while pushing the sled as fast as you can

4.   Be sure to keep your spine straight

Resistance Training

An effective and strength-building activity to add in addition to your HIIT routine is resistance training or weightlifting. When many people think of resistance training, they think of bodybuilding, which is not the same thing. Bodybuilding may be a fascinating sport, but it isn't true exercise, nor is it healthy. Body builders actually *damage* their muscle fibers in the course of trying to overdevelop them by training to failure. Healthy resistance training builds strength by only training to *fatigue*. Training to fatigue is when you can no longer complete any additional *repetitions*. Training to failure is when you can no longer complete any additional *sets*. Remember, repetitions comprise sets.

> *Healthy resistance training tones and challenges the muscles but allows ample recovery time. There are many benefits to resistance training, including: stronger bones, increased strength, healthy muscles that are less prone to injury, increased muscle mass, balanced hormone levels, and looking good. Increasing muscle mass also increases your caloric needs since muscle requires more calories than fat. This allows you to eat more during the over-eating phase without gaining any fat.*

Healthy resistance training can be done on machines or with free weights. This can be completed in less than one hour and allows for a one to two minute rest between each exercise. Resistance training can be done every other day three to four times per week, perhaps alternating with your HIIT days, If you do perform your resistance training on the same day as your HIIT, perform the HIIT first and allow at least one hour of rest before resistance training.

Resistance training will require some equipment or a gym membership. The first rule of exercise is to follow proper form, which is very important because it will keep you from getting hurt. Exercising to be healthier doesn't make much sense if you get hurt.

Types of Muscles

The muscles of the body are different in size and composition, so to make things simple, we will divide them into categories by muscle fiber concentration. When we perform resistance training, we are targeting the II b muscle fibers.

The Larger Muscles (Quads, Hamstrings, Calves, Chest, Trapezium, and Back)

The large muscles respond well to resistance training. They contain a lot of II b muscle fibers. They also tend to need greater recovery time. Generally, exercising them every ten to fourteen days is adequate. Choose two to four different exercises for each muscle group.

- The quads are the muscles in front of the thigh. Typical exercises include squats and leg presses.

- The hamstrings are the muscles in the back of the thigh. Typical exercises include leg curls.

- The calves are the muscles in the back of the leg. Typical exercises include calf raises.

- The chest muscles are in the front of the torso. Typical exercises include bench and dumbbell presses.

- The Trapezium muscles are located to the sides of the neck. Typical exercises include shoulder shrugs.

- The back muscles consist primarily of the rhomboids and the latissimus dorsi. Typical exercises include lat pull downs and seated rows.

The Smaller Muscles (Bicep, Triceps, Shoulder, Forearms)

The smaller muscles respond well, but need to be trained a little more often. They contain a fair amount of II b muscle fibers. Generally, once per week is adequate. Choose two to four different exercises for each muscle group.

- The bicep muscles are located in the front of the arm. Typical exercises include curls.

- The tricep muscles are located in the back of the arm. Typical exercises include tricep extensions.

- The shoulder muscles are located where the arm meets the torso. Typical exercises include front, side and rear raises.

- The forearm muscles are located in the front and back of the forearm. Typical exercises include wrist curls and extensions.

The Core Muscles (Abdominals, Oblique, Back Extensors, Hip Flexors)

The core muscles respond very well to body weight, or very light weight. They have relatively few II b muscle fibers. They also recover very well, so they can be trained more often. The most efficient time to perform your core exercises is in between your other resistance exercise sets. This ensures that you allow ample time for your muscles to recover between other resistance sets, and you don't have to schedule a separate core routine. The core muscle exercises should be done at a slow speed. Generally, twenty repetitions are adequate, and if it is no longer a challenge with body weight, some light weight can be added. Also, when performing your other exercises, keep your core tight by concentrating on flexing your abdominals for some added isometric core training.

A Sample Routine:

Week	Day 1	Day 2	Day 3
1	Hamstrings, Biceps, Forearms	Chest, Triceps	Quads, Shoulder, Forearms
2	Back, Biceps	Calves, Triceps, Forearms	Chest, Shoulder
3	Hamstrings, Biceps, Forearms	Back, Triceps	Quads, Shoulder, Forearms
4	Chest, Biceps	Calves, Triceps, Forearms	Back, Shoulder

It is very important to balance your training. For example, if you do three chest exercises, you should do three back exercises.

How Many Sets and Reps

A repetition is the movement of the weight from the start position through the exercise to the end point and then back to the starting point. Going from the start to end point is called the positive phase and should be done to a count of two. At the end point, there should be a very short half-second pause. The return from the end point back to the start point is called the negative phase and should be done to a count of four. There should be a half-second pause at the start point, before starting the next rep.

The timing and pauses ensure that you keep proper form and that your muscles are actually moving the weight, instead of gravity or momentum.

Four to eight repetitions will improve strength and size. Six to ten repetitions will improve strength, size and endurance. Eight to twelve repetitions will improve size and endurance. Groups of repetitions are called sets. For most exercises, three sets are sufficient. Normally, for healthy resistance training, three sets of eight repetitions are done for each exercise. I like to perform three exercises for one of the large muscles, followed by three exercises for one of the smaller muscles, with five core exercises done in between. That can be very time consuming and not as effective as we would like. Luckily, you can replace the three sets with *one drop down set* to make your resistance training even more efficient and effective.

Drop Down Sets

Drop down sets allow you to perform the above workouts in thirty minutes instead of an hour and actually get more results.

Let's assume that you would normally use fifty pounds for a particular exercise, such as dumbbell presses, when doing the standard three sets of eight reps. If you repeat that for six exercises, the amount of time quickly adds up. Another problem is that the first set is much easier than the third, and the last set ends before your muscles are fully fatigued. Using a drop down set, you can combine all three sets into one three-step set. First, because the first set is easier, you'll need to increase the weight. Try to add five to ten percent of the weight in increments that are available for the particular equipment you are using.

Here is a sample of a drop down set, using as an example your fifty pounds for three sets of eight reps. Instead of starting with fifty pounds, start with a fifty five pound weight and perform as many reps as you can. Perhaps that would be eight reps with fifty-five pounds, but perform as many as you can. Immediately remove five pounds and continue with fifty pounds and perform as many reps as you can. Let's say that would be an additional six reps with fifty pounds. Change the weight immediately to forty-five pounds and perform as many reps as you can. In this example, you did six reps with forty-five pounds. You performed a total of twenty reps over three sets with only minimal rest.

Drop Set	Weight	Reps
1	55lbs	8 (as many as possible)
2	50lbs	6 (as many as possible)
3	45lbs	6 (as many as possible)

A drop down set starts with a slightly heavier weight than you would normally use, then drops the weight down two times. By doing this, you average slightly more work per rep that you do with regular sets. An added benefit is that you engage more of the muscle fibers by varying the weight and reps in addition to doing them in much less time.

When Do I Increase the Weight?

How much weight you do is actually irrelevant, it is just a way of keeping track of your progress. Start with the minimal weight available. Increase the weight only when you are ready. If you didn't perform your reps with proper form or you are trying to impress yourself or others, that is not only dangerous, it is counterproductive to being healthy.

If you choose to do the standard method of three sets of eight reps, when you are able to perform ten reps on the last two sets for two consecutive workouts, you are ready to increase the weight five to ten percent during the next workout.

If you choose to do drop down sets, the total number of reps that you can perform over the entire drop down sets will determine if you can raise the weight five to ten percent. If you can perform twenty repetitions or more in total over the three drop down sets for two consecutive workouts, you can increase the weight.

Be honest with yourself. If you didn't have proper form, proper control of the weight, or just don't feel like you are ready, stay at the weight you have. There is no need to rush to increase it. If you are stuck at a weight and can't increase it, try decreasing the weight by twenty percent and then work your way back up.

Q. I have bad knees, what can I do?

A. If you have weak joints, including knees, hips, back or shoulders, or any musculoskeletal problems not related to trauma, these are often caused by weak muscles and/or activities that are performed improperly. Getting an evaluation to assess weak/injured muscles and joints, as well as the proper therapy, might be necessary before starting an exercise program.

Cardio/Endurance Training

Most so-called "cardio," such as running and cycling, are really sports. These are fun, recreational activities that many people enjoy, but as discussed above, they are not true exercise. You may enjoy cardio exercises, but you should still perform HIIT for a strong heart and lungs and to increase your metabolism.

If you have a lot of body fat to lose, you can add some endurance training after your HIIT to burn some additional calories. Jogging and biking are effective endurance activities. Just be careful about doing too much, as it will increase your hunger.

Warm ups, Cool Downs, and Stretching

There still seems to be some confusion about the difference between warming up and stretching that needs to be cleared up.

Warming up is done by performing a low intensity activity such as walking for a couple of minutes before exercising. The purpose is to make sure that there is good blood flow to the muscles so they don't cramp. You should always warm up before exercising.

Cooling down is actually more similar to warming up: you cool down by performing a low intensity exercise for a couple of minutes after exercising. A cool-down period allows your body to use up waste products so they aren't left in the muscles.

There are two types of stretching: active stretching, which is beneficial, and passive stretching, which is not. When muscles are weak or over used, they may become tight. They no longer contract and relax properly. The best way to describe this is to think of a rope. When you tie a knot into the rope, the rope becomes shorter. In a muscle, a knot also makes it shorter, and you notice a decrease in your range of motion. Your first thought might be to stretch it out. Initially, this might feel better, but just as if you pull on the ends of the rope the knot becomes tighter, so does your muscle. That is called passive (or static) stretching.

Passive stretching forcibly lengthens the muscle by pulling on it to the normal end range of motion. An example would be touching your toes to stretch your hamstring. Because passive stretching causes the muscle to reflexively contract against the pull, there is really no need to do any passive stretching. In fact, passive stretching can actually tear IIb muscle fibers, causing knots in the muscles, especially when done past the normal range of motion. So, it can sometimes be responsible for increasing the risk of injury, as opposed to the common misconception of lowering the risk of injury.

Active stretching is when you contract the muscles opposite to the muscles you want to stretch for ten seconds. Your body can't contract opposite muscles at the same time. So, by contracting the opposite muscle, you are allowing the tight muscle to relax and lengthen as much as possible. An example would be bending your foot up and lifting your leg, without assistance, straight out in front of you to stretch the hamstring. You would usually perform that for a count of ten and repeat it three times. Active stretching can be done any time that a muscle is sore, cramping, or feels tight. You can also massage the muscle to help with blood flow and reduce trigger points zones and knots that develop in the muscles.

Sleep, Rest, and Recovery

Your body needs time to heal itself and prepare for activity. Planning for restful times is just as important as planning for activity.

During sleep, the body heals, repairs, regulates, burns fat, and cleans itself. It also allows your mind to sort and store all the information it needs to process. Planning adequate sleep time is a very important part of a health plan. How much time varies from person to person, but eight hours is a good starting point.

When you are sleeping, the body can replenish used glycogen stores.

When you are exercising, periods of recovery allow the body to stabilize your heart rate, breathing rate, blood sugar levels, hormone levels, and catch up on ATP production. Your body has enough ATP for about an hour of resistance training or two hours of endurance training. After that, it may start to break down muscle for fuel.

When to Exercise

Just like with eating, *when you exercise* is also important. HIIT training is best performed first thing in the morning, before eating, to maximize the fat burning effect. Resistance training is also more effective early in the day. Since we are inherently nocturnal eaters, it goes against our natural body rhythm to exercise in the evening.

Post-Workout Recovery Meal

About a half hour after exercising, your muscle glycogen is depleted and your insulin receptors are peaked. This is the time to use non-fiber, starch carbohydrates to your advantage. A normal post-workout recovery meal would be ten to thirty grams of protein and ten to thirty grams of non-fiber, starch carbohydrates, depending on how much exercise you completed. For example, ten grams protein and ten grams non-fiber, starch carbs would be ideal after a HIIT workout of three sets. Twenty grams of each would be ideal after a HIIT workout of six sets. If you worked out for nine sets of HIIT or resistance/endurance training, then thirty grams of protein and thirty grams of non-fiber, starch carbs would be appropriate.

Sports drinks might seem like a good idea, but the amount of sugar carbs per serving is usually too high, so I don't recommend them.

Q. I get tired, dizzy, or light-headed during or after my workout. How can I prevent this?

A. One reason this happens may be due to the fact that your body is still not efficient at burning fat. Alternatively, it might be that you are too lean. In either case, your blood sugar is getting too low.

If you are getting tired during your workout, try eating some non-fiber, starch carbs *the night before* during your over-eating phase. Try adding non-fiber, starch carbs in increments of 10g, until you have enough energy for your workouts. However, if you are very lean or do very calorie intensive workouts, you might need a pre-workout meal.

Start with 10g or protein and 10g of non-fiber, starch carbs. If you are trying to lose fat weight, do not eat before or during your workout, just drink water.

If you are getting tired after your workout, you need to eat a post-workout recovery meal. My normal recommendation is thirty grams of protein, followed by thirty grams of non-fiber, starch carbs.

How Muscle Tone Impacts Weight

As a Chiropractic Neuromyologist, I have been working with
muscle tone related problems throughout my career. There is an
interesting connection between the tone of muscles in the neck
and base of the skull and weight problems. In order to understand
this connection, you must first understand the sphenoid sinus and
its role in human health. The sphenoid sinus is located inside of
the skull and has a powerful effect on the pituitary and
hypothalamus, which are glands located in the brain. Together,
these glands control the ANS, autonomic nervous system. This
system includes the neuroendocrine system, which affects your
entire body chemistry.

The pituitary gland is an extension of the hypothalamus and
must operate at a slightly lower temperature than the rest of the
brain. The primary role of the sphenoid sinus is to cool the
pituitary, much like the radiator of a car helps to cool the engine.
The way in which it does this is by releasing a clear fluid that
evaporates and cools the sinus cavity.

There are several factors that affect the sphenoid sinus, one of
which is weather. The linings of the sinus react to changes in
humidity and pressure. This affects the rate at which the clear fluid
evaporates. When humidity and air pressure are low, the membranes
in the sinus tend to sponge up fluid and begin to swell. Airplane
travel can also affect pressure changes and irritate the sinus. When
muscles at the base of the skull and neck lose their normal tone, in
effect becoming tighter, which can occur from a number of factors,
a sphenoid sinus reflex nerve can become irritated. Depending upon
the levels of irritation, histamine can be released, which stimulates
the linings of the sinus to overproduce fluid. The swollen
membranes around the sinus openings then shut and pressure builds
up inside of the sinus. This is usually not recognized on an x-ray

because many times there is no infection present, and it is the pus caused by an infection that is seen on a study.

Now, when the sphenoid sinus becomes blocked, the ability to cool the pituitary and hypothalamus is lost, which can lead to dysfunction of these glands. This swelling pressure can cause the bone of the sinus to press into the pituitary and base of the hypothalamus, which can interfere with the function of the autonomic nervous system. An irritated sinus can lead to excessive amounts of histamine being released, which is responsible for inflammations, irritation, and a host of symptoms that range from allergies, depression, and even aggravating other existing illnesses. In particular, pressure and interference with the pituitary can result in an overproduction of ADH, anti-diuretic hormone, and a lack of production of hormones that control sugar metabolism. Those hormones are thyrotropin and ACTH, adrenocorticotropic hormone. This cycle of imbalance can lead to a person getting bloated and fat!

The way in which I have addressed this issue is by using a specific type of muscle massage on the neck and base of the skull. This type of massage involves two different methods. One is by a machine which delivers a specific type of stimulation known as percussion, and the other type is by fingertip, which cross strokes over the muscles with a specific type of movement and tension. These types of actions generate a strong biological nerve response that activates muscle feedback nerves and then stimulate areas of the brain known as the cerebellum. The results of this action causes muscles to relax their excessive tone, hypertonic spasm, and allow a full capacity of blood and a host of other healing fluids and chemicals to clean and improve the affected muscles, leading to a stronger and healthier nerve response. In conclusion, healthy neck muscles will support a body chemistry which is in line with a slimmer body.

How Sound & Radio Waves Can Trigger Fat Loss & Create Tighter Skin

I have discovered the amazing benefits of using sound waves to release tight, stubborn fat from the body. Ultrasound waves have historically been used to visualize fetal development, structures of the body, and even break up kidney stones, known as lithotripsy. Ultrasound waves are now being used to open up fat cell membranes in order to release stubborn, tucked away fat, safely and in total comfort with no downtime! This is something I have been using in my practice, and the results have been quite impressive. Once introducing these sound waves, the fat is able to be released into the body's interstitial fluid. In this state, the fat is presented to the body's metabolism for processing, instead of staying hidden away. Taking it one step further, we introduce a Radio wave (known as RF or Radio Frequency) once the sound wave treatment is completed. This works on the fat that has just been released and melts it down into its more basic components—glycerol and fatty acids. The body then naturally transports the contents through the lymphatic and vascular systems to the liver, where it is processed and eliminated naturally. The radio waves even take it one step further. While it acts to melt fat, it simultaneously activates fibroblasts under the skin's surface, which causes new collagen to form. As a result, the skin becomes tighter over that region. There are two aspects of this tightening: one is an immediate contractile and smoothing effect to the skin; the second is the true collagen growth, which occurs over a course of approximately nine to sixteen weeks, which is the longer term effects of the tightening.

Here are some examples of before and after pictures of clients who followed the protocol:

Before   **After 4 Treatments**

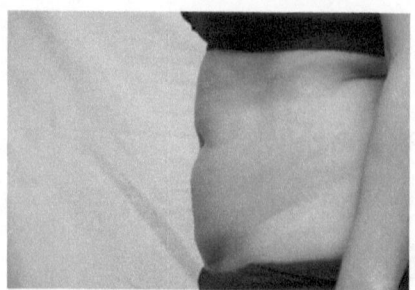
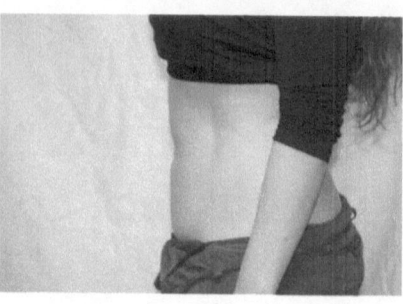

Before   **After 9 Treatments**

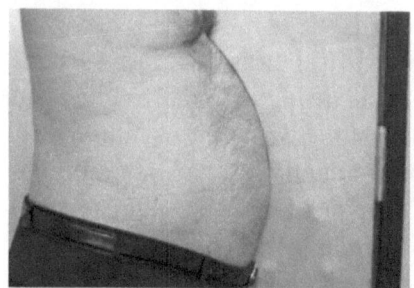
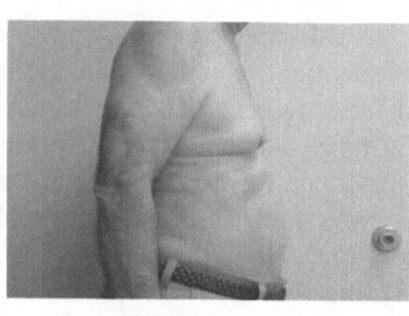

Before   **After 5 Treatments**

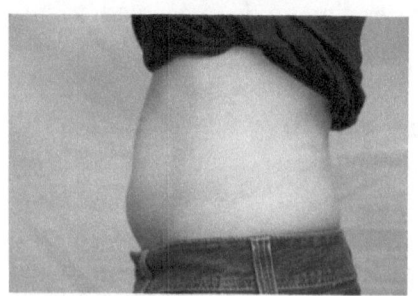
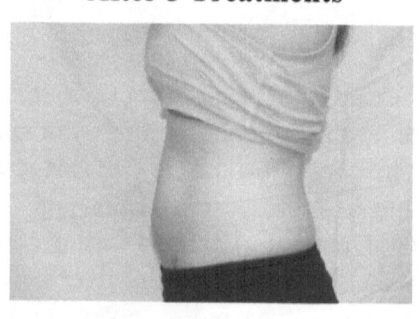

Before   **After 6 Treatments**

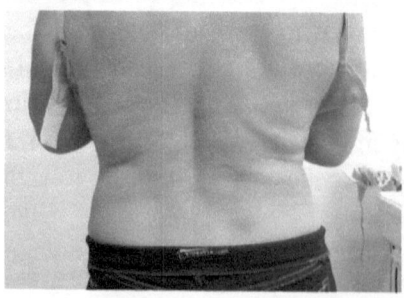
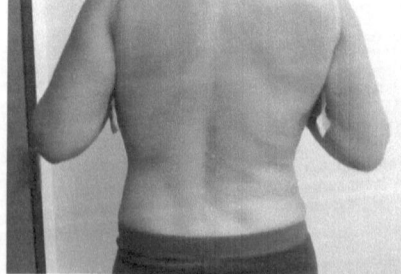

My clients have asked me if the fat comes back after a while. The answer is no if you follow the right kind of eating habits, which will help to detoxify your system as well as bring your hormonal levels in balance. Eating is a hormonal event and absolutely influences fat content. If a person continues to throw their blood sugar out of control by creating insulin spikes and ultimately insulin resistance and/or eating improperly in the wrong timing, sure, the fat will tend to redevelop over time. Remember, activate your fat burning hormones (glucagon, growth hormone, insulin like growth factor, testosterone, adrenaline and thyroid), not your fat storing hormones (insulin, cortisol and estrogen).

In this process, fat cells are not being removed as they are when someone undergoes liposuction, lipo freezing, or other similar procedures. Simply, it is like emptying a garbage can of fat. It is healthier to leave the fat cells intact, and it also prevents fat from being distributed to unusual areas such as around the knees, neck, etc. should you regain it. The wonderful thing about this treatment option is that it not only can jumpstart the fat dissolving and slenderizing process, it can also help to remove fat that might never have been addressed by the body's metabolism, not to the mention the benefits of the skin tightening effect.

Biofeedback for Stress Reduction

Stress, whether it's from physical, chemical or emotional sources, can act to create distress within us, disrupting our natural cycles of healthy function. With excessive stress, our sleep, digestion, focus and fat burning ability can become impaired. One of the stress hormones is cortisol and as we learned earlier, it is also one of our fat storing hormones. Sustaining high amounts of unresolved stress, whether conscious or unconscious, over time acts to suppress our ability to burn fat and maintain optimal function. I have found that biofeedback therapy can be a highly effective aid in helping to restore mind body balance and further aid in fat burning.

Making the Most of This Book

Now that you know how diet and exercise affect the body and how to start a plan, we need to review, clarify, and answer some lingering questions. This section will help you take the information you just learned and put it into action. If you still have questions even after reading this section, please visit my website:

www.secretsofslender.com

You can send me questions there and share information with other readers.

The Principles

The following are the top ten principle lessons from this book:

- All food has an aging effect. Make the most optimal food choice when possible.
- *When* you eat, is as important as *what* you eat. Try to eat only live foods during the day.
- It is perfectly acceptable to have short periods of under-eating and over-eating, as long as the overall quantity is balanced.
- Drink filtered or spring water only when you are thirsty; do not attempt to overhydrate.
- Try to limit the amount of insulin your body releases during the day by eating starch carbs only during the carb friendly times and avoiding sugar.
- Choose live foods first.
- Schedule times for foods that you want or crave.

- Use High Intensity Interval Training (HIIT) to build your heart and lungs.

- Proper form and timing are the most important parts of an exercise plan.

- Drop down sets can make your resistance training more time efficient & effective.

- Only increase the weight if you are ready.

The 5 Misconceptions:

Misconception #1: Eating at night will cause weight gain.

It has long be touted that eating late in the day is the worst time to eat because the body slows down and will become prone to weight gain. I can see how this notion might make some sense; however, it is not true. There haven't been any conclusive studies or evidence to demonstrate that eating meals late in the day will cause you to gain fat. There are other variables which have a major impact on fat gain/loss, which include the sugar producing potential of a meal (glycemic index), the frequency eating, timing of meals as well as the volume of food consumed during particular meals of the day. Humans are inherently night eaters, and planning the main meal to occur at dinnertime can be highly advantageous in burning fat as well as highly rewarding. We have in internal clock that we are inherently programmed to function around, known as the circadian clock. This clock dictates that we are active during the day and relax at night. That inner clock is directly influenced by our nervous system. There are two parts of our nervous system that play into this clock: the sympathetic nervous system (SNS)—high alert, focused, active and fight/flight mechanism for survival; and the parasympathetic nervous system (PSNS), which activates digestion, relaxation and sleep. It is at rest during the night that the human body is able to digest and utilize nutrients as opposed to the stress related periods during the day and all of its activities. It is during the night when growth hormone (GH) reaches its peak level. Growth hormone builds muscle and bone and burns fat.

Misconception #2: Eating fat will make you fat.

Thinking on a simple level that eating fat will turn into just that is another common notion that at the surface might seem to be true. Humans do better on certain types of fats such as nuts, seeds, high quality eggs, and olive oil as opposed to the fats from processed foods. Fat is a high quality fuel for the body, and the muscle is the organ that creates the largest demand for fat. Fat plays a major role in the body such as in regulating blood pressure, inflammation, stress reactions, building and maintaining cell membranes, aiding the function of nerves, maintaining the integrity of the immune system, producing hormones, and being a source of fuel. Choose high-quality fats and you will get the most out of this critical fuel.

Misconception #3: Carbohydrates are the body's enemy and will make you fat.

Carbohydrates play a critical role in maintaining body functions, which go beyond energy production. While it is true that eating particular types of carbohydrates that boil down to an appreciable amount of sugar, such as processed foods, cookies, candies, cakes, sodas, etc, will cause insulin to spike up and can ultimately be stored as fat. However, other types of carbohydrates that are "non-starchy," such as vegetables, certain fruits, and salads, do not spike insulin and provide a wonderful balance to the diet. Carbohydrates also complete a complex chemical process in the composition of growth hormone, insulin growth factor, and sex steroid hormones, all of which are critical to our wellness and longevity. Staying on a diet of carbohydrate restriction will lead to metabolic decline and loss of health.

Misconception #4: Breakfast is the most important meal of the day.

Did you know that eating a big breakfast shuts down your weight loss cycle? I know how many sources over the years have claimed that a breakfast is the most important meal of the day. The morning time is when your body is in self-cleaning mode, also known as the detoxification cycle. This is the cycle when your body's survival mechanism, from the sympathetic nervous system, is activated and generating energy for the day as well as resisting fatigue and stress. This is when energy should come from burning our stored fat. This is allowed to occur as long as you don't pull your body down by consuming a heavy meal. Does this mean that you should not eat anything in the morning? No, you absolutely can eat; however, your food choices here are critical and should be live foods in low quantity. The most important meals of the day are the post-workout recovery meal and dinner.

Misconception #5: Counting calories will help me to control weight and lose fat.

Calorie counting has been integrated in some of the most popular weight-loss systems today. It is the method in which they control food and energy intake. The problem is that this method fails to create a long term, sustainable benefit for staying lean as well as maintaining health. The human organism is a dynamic one, and we use and regulate fuel based upon fluctuating conditions in physical activity, environmental conditions, and other stressors. This means that at times we may need fewer or more calories, depending upon what is happening in life. A low-calorie diet promotes a lower metabolic rate, and since calorie counting is based upon a fixed basal metabolic rate (BMR), it fails to account for real life demands and changing conditions. It's also true that not all calories are the same. A calorie coming from a sugar food will more likely trigger a fat gain as opposed to calories coming from other fuel sources. Timing is another important factor for calorie consumption. Carbohydrate consumption right after a workout would have great benefits as opposed to consuming it prior to a workout. This tends to trigger a release of cortisol, which has harmful effects, as well as storage of belly fat. Calorie restriction also leads to lower body temperature, loss of libido, decline in sex hormones, and loss of overall vigor, potency, fertility, and performance.

Tracking Your Progress

Numbers are an important aspect of health. They allow us to determine certain levels of health and track progress. The catch is determining which numbers are "normal" and using the numbers in the correct context.

Body weight is an important number. However, using it to track health and progress can be flawed. For example, many people weigh the same now as they did five to ten years prior, but they tend to look very different and are in different health.

Let's say we are presented with two people: A and B. Both are thirty-five-year-old men, 5'9" tall and 160 pounds. The A might be muscular, and the B might be slightly overweight. Using just the total weight as a basis, you wouldn't know which was healthy or unhealthy. This is the first problem with using body weight as a parameter.

Let's say A stops exercising and maintains his eating habits while B decides to stop eating non-fiber, starch carbs. Six months later, they both weigh 150 pounds. What happened?

Since A stopped exercising, he lost muscle; while B stopped eating non-fiber, starch carbs and lost fat.

Now B starts exercising and builds some muscle. His weight goes back up to 160 pounds. He's right back where he started, but he is eating better and exercising. He is in much better health and probably looks great.

Just like cholesterol, it isn't enough to know the total. If you only look at the total when you start exercising, you might gain a few pounds of muscle and your lack of weight loss might discourage you. A healthy person doesn't seek to lose *weight*; they seek to lose *fat*.

> *The correct way to track this aspect of health is by measuring body fat, which can easily tell you if your weight is healthy.*

Thanks to modern science, the cumbersome and difficult task of measuring body fat is now as simple as stepping on a scale. New high-tech scales from manufacturers like Tanita[1] can measure your weight and body fat percentage in seconds, with a high degree of accuracy. The better scales reveal many details about your metabolism, such as total weight, body fat percent, metabolic age, visceral fat, muscle weight, water percent, bone weight, basal metabolic rate, and more.

---

[1] I mention Tanita only because they are widely available, but there are many other brands that may be as good or even better.

Take your total body weight and multiply it by your percent body fat. That is your fat weight, and this is the number you want to track. In my own case, while my weight remained constant, I went from sixteen percent body fat to eight percent body fat. I lost ten pounds of fat, but gained ten pounds of muscle! If total weight was my only method of tracking my progress, I would not have been successful.

Initially, A's body fat was around fifteen percent and B's about twenty-one percent. Even though A lost ten pounds, his body fat increased by eighteen percent, so we know that he gained three pounds of fat and lost thirteen pounds of water/muscle. B went from thirty-four pounds of fat down to twenty-nine pounds yet, in total, he still weighed exactly the same! It's easy to see how valuable this measurement is.

If you don't have a body fat scale or don't want to use one, waist size is a much better indicator of health than your body weight.

Here are the standard body fat ranges:

Female Age	Under fat or athlete	Healthy	Less Healthy	Unhealthy
20 to 39	0% to 21%	22 to 33%	34 to 39%	40% and up
40 to 59	0% to 23%	24 to 34%	35 to 40%	41% and up
60 to 79	0% to 24%	25 to 36%	37 to 42%	43% and up

Male Age	Under fat or athlete	Healthy	Less Healthy	Unhealthy
20 to 39	0% to 8%	9 to 20%	21 to 25%	26% and up
40 to 59	0% to 11%	12 to 22%	23 to 28%	29% and up
60 to 79	0% to 13%	14 to 25%	26 to 30%	31% and up

Also note that there are other parameters to be aware of to help measure your overall improvement. These include energy levels, sleep quality, amount of sleep, cravings, overall digestion, and inches lost.

Food Choices

With so many foods available, it would be impossible for me list them all. But I've listed most common foods, and a few uncommon choices, and placed them into the category they best fit.

This is a good time to mention the issues with "natural food." Just because a food is packaged as "natural" doesn't mean it's true. There are a few things you need to be aware of before consuming food.

1. Chemical sprays, insecticides, and pesticides. These chemicals have been used to reduce the amount of crop loss. Consuming these products, which are usually labeled "conventional," will only counteract your efforts in loosing fat and getting healthier. I recommend staying away from these products as much as you can.

2. Chemicals added to foods that make them addictive. One main one is MSG, monosodium glutamate. It blocks the sensation of feeling satisfied from your meal, and it enhances your food by sensitizing your taste buds. It ultimately fools your brain and causes you to eat more. Steer clear of this one.

3. Antibiotics have been used in order to make animals grow larger and prevent infections. Could this be responsible for the super strains of bacteria?

4. Growth hormones are used to primarily cause animals to get big quickly. This leads to greater profits within the food industry.

I choose organic foods, which are devoid of these chemicals; I recommend you do as well.

Best Live Foods

These foods provide optimal nutrition and can be eaten in moderation at any time during the day.

Seeds, Nuts, and Nut Butters:

Almonds	Pistachios	Sesame Tahini
Brazil nuts	Poppy	Sunflower
Cashews	Pumpkin	Walnuts
Pecans	Sesame	

(Preferably raw and unsalted)

Fish and Seafood:

Crab	Oysters	Scallops
Halibut	Salmon	Shrimp
Herring	Sardines	Trout
Lobster	Mackerel	Tuna

(If canned, preferably in olive oil or water)

Meats, Protein:

Bear	Organic	Veggie Burgers
Buffalo	Pheasant	Venison
Chicken	Poultry	
Eggs	Protein Powder*	

(Preferably Wild Or Pastured, Flax Or Grass Fed)
(*Egg or Whey, look for no added sugar or artificial sweeteners)

Dairy:

Cheddar	Cream Cheese	Provolone
Colby	Havarti	Raw Milk
Cottage Cheese	Monterey Jack	

(Dairies sometimes add sugar to non- or low-fat for flavor, so watch for added sugar content)

Raw Oils:

Cod Liver Oil

Flax Oil

Hemp Oil

Olive Oil

Greens and vegetables:

Artichoke Hearts

Arugula

Asparagus

Bamboo Shoots

Beet

Bell Peppers

Bok Choy

Broccoli

Brussels Sprouts

Cabbage

Cauliflower

Celery

Chard

Chives

Collards

Cucumbers

Eggplant

Garlic

Green Peppers

Hot Peppers

Kale

Leaf Lettuce

Leeks

Mustard

Okra

Onions

Pickles

Radish

Radishes

Red Peppers

Romaine Lettuce

Scallions

Snow Pea Pods

Spinach

Sprouts

String Beans

Summer Squash

Turnip

Turnips

Water Chestnuts

Zucchini

(Fresh or no-salt frozen, unsweetened)

Mushrooms:

Button

Oyster

Portabella

Shitake

Seaweeds:

Dulse

Hijiki

Kombu

Nori

Fruits:

Apricot	Date (Deglet)	Pineapple
Apples	Grapefruit	Prune
Avocados	Guava	Raspberries
Blackberries	Kiwi	Star Fruit
Boysenberries	Lemon	Strawberries
Cantaloupe	Lime	Tangerine
Cherries	Mandarin	Tomatoes
Clementine	Olives	
Cranberries	Passion Fruit	

(One serving = one small piece whole fruit or one half cup, fresh, not canned)

Condiments and Spices:

Basil	Fennel	Oregano
Black Pepper	Garlic	Tamari
Capers	Ginger	Turmeric
Cayenne Pepper	Garam Masala	
Cumin	Mustard	

Sweeteners:

Stevia	Xylitol

(Be careful as they tend to increase hunger)

I find that apples, raw nuts, avocados, eggs, vegetables, sprouts, bee pollen & plain greek yogurt are some of my favorite foods for the under-eating phase. Experiment and see what works best for you.

Best Foods for Over-Eating Phases

These foods provide adequate nutrition. They are fine to consume during your over-eating phase. They also can be eaten during the under-eating phase, but in small quantities.

Meat:

Beef   Lamb

(Pastured, leaner cuts)

Dairy:

Cream   Milk (Whole)
Ghee   Yogurt (Plain)

Smaller Beans:

Adzuki   Mung
Black   Navy
Lentil

Cooking Oils:

Coconut Oil   Olive Oil

Vegetables (including the greens and vegetables from the previous section):

Carrots   Parsnips   Peas

Fruits:

Banana   Honeydew   Papaya
Blueberries   Nectarine   Peach
Date (Medjool)   Orange

(One serving = one small piece whole fruit or one half cup, fresh, not canned)

Non-Fiber Carbohydrates:

Brown Rice   Whole Grain Breads
Dark Breads   Whole Grain Oatmeal

(Best eaten after live foods, in moderation)

Q. Is dark chocolate good for you?

A. The darker the chocolate—seventy percent or higher—the healthier it is. A small amount is best, about one ounce at any time. Milk chocolate, or dark that is less than seventy percent, should be reserved for your evening snack, if at all. I recommend ninety to one hundred percent chocolate as it is a very healthy choice, but it can take some getting used to. However, if you only take a small piece and let it melt in your mouth instead of chewing it, it is more palatable. Follow it with a sip of full-bodied red wine to bring out the flavors. I regularly enjoy ninety percent dark chocolate throughout the week, after my evening meal.

A Note About Nuts

Eating an ample quantity of raw nuts is important. Some people could be allergic to nuts or tend to experience bloating, gas, and heaviness after eating them. This bloating is usually due to the enzyme inhibitors that are inherently in nuts. If we do not inactivate these enzyme inhibitors before consuming them, our pancreas has to work much harder to digest them, essentially releasing many more of its own enzymes. A pancreas that is stressed will cause digestion to slow down and lead to bloating, etc. If this happens over an extended period of time, you can lose your enzyme reserves and have a harder time digesting foods. These symptoms are often confused with having food allergies but are really the result of a lack of enzymes in our own body. The best way to deal with this issue is to germinate your nuts and seeds. Simply do the following:

1. Soak the nuts and seeds in a covered glass or metal container filled with filtered water over the course of twelve hours; overnight is best.

2. In the morning, drain off all of the fluid, which contains the enzyme inhibitors; you will see how the fluid appears murky. Then rinse the nuts and seeds.

3. Allow them to air dry in a strainer. When complete, keep them refrigerated. Only soak the volume of nuts and seeds you plan to consume over the following five

to six days. Soaking them causes them to activate into a livened state, and foods that are alive are vulnerable to spoiling.

4.   Your nuts and seeds are now a fantastic food to consume, and as a result of removing all of the enzyme inhibitors, you have just avoided placing considerable stress on your digestive system.

5.   Again, store what you don't eat in a glass container and make sure to keep them refrigerated.

Foods to Limit

These foods provide only fair nutrition. They are fine to consume in moderation during the over-eating phase, especially after eating foods from the previous two sections.

Larger Beans:

Chick Peas	Lima	Peanuts
Garbanzo	Peanut Butter	Pinto

Corn:

Canned	Cornbread	Popped
Cob	Frozen	Tortillas

Fruits:

Figs	Mango	Persimmon
Grapes	Pear	Watermelon

(One serving = one small piece whole fruit or one half cup, fresh, not canned)

Artificial Sweeteners*:

Acesulfame	Isomalt	Sorbitol
Potassium	Maltodextrin	Sucralose
Erythritol	Mannitol	

(*Although artificial sweeteners are not consumed for nutrition, but for taste, I added them here because they are so prevalent.)

Other:

Butter	Pizza
Egg Pasta	Pork
Honey	Rice Pasta
Ice Cream	Salt
Milk*	Whole Wheat Pasta

(*Fat Free, Skim, 1%, 2%, Pasteurized)

Foods to Avoid Completely (Dead Foods)

These foods provide poor nutrition. Ideally, you would never eat anything in this section. However, if you think you must eat these, you should limit the quantity as much as possible and restrict them to the end of the over-eating phase.

Oils:

Corn	Margarine	Shortening
Hydrogenated	Peanut	Sunflower
Lite Butter	Processed Oils	

(All foods containing hydrogenated oils)

Chips:

Cheese Curls	Corn	Potato

(Baked are better than fried)

Condiments:

BBQ Sauce
Ketchup

Mayonnaise
Worcestershire

(Especially if they contain hydrogenated fats and sugar)

Artificial Sweeteners:

Alitame
Aspartame
Brazzein
Curculin
Glucin
Glycerol
Glycyrrhizin
Hydrogenated Starch
Hydrolysates
Lactitol
Maltitol

Malto-Oligosaccharide
Neohesperidin
Dihydrochalcone
Neotame
Nutrasweet
Nutrinova
Saccharin
Sweet 'N Low
Tagatose
Twinsweet

Natural Sweeteners: (used as additives)

Dextrose
Fructose
Molasses

Sucrose
Sugars
Syrups

Turbinado

(Especially high- fructose corn syrup)

Sweets:

Cakes
Candies
Cookies
Diet Soda

Dried Fruits
Fruit Juice
Soda
Sports Drinks

Sweets
Sweetened Tea

Preservatives: (found in most processed foods)

BHA (Butylated
Hydroxyanisole)
BHT (Butylated
Hydrozyttoluene)

Propyl Gallate
Sodium Nitrite

Food Additives:

Monosodium Glutamate
(MSG)
Olestra

Potassium Bromate
Trans Fats

Other:

American cheese
Bacon
Dry Packaged Breakfast
Cereal
Flavored Yogurt
French Fries
Fried Foods

Hot Dogs
Pork Products
Powdered Milk
Processed Cold Cut Meats
White Bread
White Potatoes
White Rice

Supplements

Although we should get all of our nutrients from our diet, there are reasons for taking additional vitamin and mineral supplements. You might not have access to high quality food, have a specific lifestyle, or illness that requires additional nutrients. Here is a list of some of the most common supplements and why you might benefit from including them. All of these are available at your local nutrition store. I highly recommend consuming a food- based vitamin as opposed to synthetic (fractional) vitamins. Fractional vitamins are cheaper to produce as well as less costly to buy, however, have no real value for our bodies and can irritate and degrade our body tissues. Check the back of the label and see if actual food is mentioned. Then check the individual ingredients and notice the amount of milligrams for each vitamin. If the vitamins are synthetic you will see the same amount of milligrams listed for each of the vitamins. If you are looking at a whole food vitamin there will be different amounts listed for each of the vitamins.

Bee pollen

I recommend that everyone consume at least a tablespoon of granulated, local bee pollen daily. Bee pollen contains *every* nutrient required by the human body, not to mention a great source of protein. There is also some expert opinion that consuming locally collected bee pollen reduces the incidence of allergic reactions to airborne pollen.

Multivitamin

A good whole-food multivitamin is inexpensive and a simple way to ensure that you have all the nutrients you need.

Omega-3 Fish Oils

Because most of us have a diet that is too low in Omega-3, which contains so many anti-inflammatory benefits, I recommend taking one of the many brands available in pill form.

Antioxidant Complex

A good antioxidant complex from natural sources will include Ascorbic acid (Vitamin C), Glutathione, Lipoic acid, Uric acid, Carotenes, Retinol (vitamin A), α-Tocopherol (vitamin E), and Ubiquinol (coenzyme Q). This will help with healing, elimination of toxins, and general health.

Zinc, Protein

These will help your body if you are a vegetarian, recovering from a surgery or serious illness, or engage in endurance sports.

Calcium, Magnesium, Iron

These supplements will especially benefit women or those with poor bone density, as well as men and women who rarely exercise. Look for chelated products, which have better absorption.

Probiotics and Acidophilus

Your "good bacteria" may be deficient if you don't eat fermented foods, have bowel issues, or have recently used antibiotics. You can supplement with probiotics or Acidophilus to rebuild them.

Glucosamine Sulfate, Chondroitin, MSM

There seem to be some conflicting studies and opinion on whether these supplements can help with arthritis. My best suggestion is that if you have arthritis, or are over forty and have a family history of arthritis, you might consider using them.

A Note About Household and Personal Care Products

Just like much of our food contains chemicals that will interfere with our hormonal and glandular systems, much of the household and personal care products are loaded with many of these chemicals as well. Everything from makeup, hairsprays, soaps, shampoos, colognes, perfumes, body lotions, moisturizers, and dish and clothing detergents contain everything from parabens to other chemicals that mimic actions of estrogen. Even our mattresses contain a boatload of chemicals! When estrogen is increased, guess what else will start to increase? That's right, fat! It's critical to remove as many influences of these chemicals from our environment as we can. Not that you have to become a fanatic; however, if you consider that what you cannot directly see can create harmful effects, both short and long term, you might want to consider using the natural alternatives that are available in many health food stores and do a great job. As you can see, it's not just a fat issue, it's a matter of not becoming a filter for these commonly used commercial chemicals, whether you are looking to become slender or not.

A Sample Daily Schedule

Here's a sample guideline and starting point for a beginner:

Breakfast: Cranberry-apple-cider-vinegar-lemon-in-water drink on an empty stomach (see Water section for mixture values), one–half cup berries or one-half grapefruit, and one-half cup of plain low-fat greek yogurt with flaxseeds or two hard boiled eggs. You can have black coffee here. I recommend no more than 1 cup of organic coffee.

HIIT or Resistance Training: Drink water before, during, and after. If your primary goal is weight loss, you should *exercise before eating*.

Post-workout recovery meal: Protein shake (see recipe) and one or two slices of Ezekiel bread with either clarified butter (ghee) or light cream cheese.

Mid-morning snack: Two tablespoons of bee pollen and one cup of raspberry zinger tea (Celestial Seasonings, all natural, caffeine-free) or an egg and an walnuts.

Late morning snack: Two ounces of cheddar cheese or a poached egg and some almonds, glass of water.

Lunch: Cranberry-apple-cider-vinegar-lemon-in-water drink, avocado salad (see recipe), and glass of water. Depending on your activity level and hunger, you might skip lunch two or three times per week.

Mid-afternoon snack: One-half cup mixed raw/unsalted nuts, glass of water, and a small apple.

Dinner: I always like to start my dinner with a big salad. I mix in organic red cabbage with other types of lettuce and greens, raw beets, peppers, salsa, sea salt, raw sauerkraut, tomatoes, olive oil, and any other vegetables I want to mix in. I like to wait about twenty minutes or so after finishing my salad before moving onto a protein. Chicken breasts and zucchini with tomato, spices, and half cup of brown rice. Keep in mind that the quantity consumed can vary on any given day, depending on your appetite. One night you might find one breast sufficient, other nights two or three.

Alternate Dinner: Salad, salmon, brown rice, and vegetables.

Alternate Dinner: Stir Fry (see recipe)

Dessert: if you did choose to schedule a dessert, this would be the best time. Try to keep the portion to a few hundred calories or less.

Evening snack: Dark chocolate and one glass of red wine.

Sample Recipes

My best suggestion for preparing meals is to experiment with spices. Once you find combinations that you like, foods take on entirely different characteristics. For example, adding combinations of capers, ginger, cumin, turmeric, sea salt, oregano, and thyme to salads and different foods makes meals take on a different taste and experience. Keep your meals interesting and exciting by substituting different foods from the lists I have provided. Take these lists with you when you go food shopping so that you will keep a consistent supply of nutrient dense foods available. Remember, do not overeat during the day; think of it as grazing with live foods. Consume your main meal at dinnertime. This is how your body will learn to rely on your own fat reserves, in addition to dietary fat, in order to bring your towards your goals and enhance your health.

Post-Workout Protein Shake

One small/medium banana

Three-fourths cup of liquid (black coffee, water, or whole milk, raw if available)

One tablespoon almond butter

Two scoops of quality protein powder, preferably whey that is Non-Denatured and chemical free

Blend together and drink after exercise.

Avocado Salad
(by varying combinations, you can reinvent this every day)

One half avocado

Protein (pick one: half-can of tuna in olive oil, or a half-cup of nuts/seeds, or chicken)

Cheese (your choice)

Onion to taste, chopped

Olive oil

Half of a tomato diced

Spices: try capers, cumin, ginger, thyme, and red pepper, to taste

Combine ingredients in bowl.

Stir Fry
(change ingredients when you want variety)

Protein (Meat or fish)

Vegetables (cut evenly)

Spices

Optional non-fiber, starch carb: one-half cup brown rice, rice noodle, egg noodle, black beans, etc.

Using high heat, add just enough oil in the wok to coat ingredients (about two tablespoons). Let the oil get hot, but not smoking, and add your chopped protein. Cook until the protein changes color. Remove the protein and set it aside.

Rinse the wok under cold water to remove anything that might burn. Return the wok to high heat and add new oil. If using garlic, sliced ginger and/or onions add them first and cook for about fifteen seconds.

Add your vegetables and cook for about two minutes while stirring.

Then add the protein back in, and any optional carb you are using. Add spices and cook for one minute.

Decoding Food Labels:

Serving Size

Pay attention to the serving size on food labels because they will often make it very small to make you think it has fewer calories or less sugar.

Calories

Calories are simply the energy contained in the food. If you are trying to lose weight, try to limit the amount of total calories to one hundred to three hundred per meal/snack. If you are lean, you may eat two hundred to five hundred calories per meal/snack. Keep in mind that any energy you consume above your immediate needs will be stored as fat.

Saturated Fat

The less saturated fat the product contains, the better. Try for zero.

Trans Fat

There is no amount of trans fat that is healthy.

Sodium (Salt)

Sodium is an important nutrient for the human body. Unfortunately, in very high quantities it can affect your health, and the average American diet is very high in sodium. The total daily intake should be between 1,000 mg and 2,000 mg. Commercial vegetable drinks like V-8 contain more than seven hundred milligrams per serving, so it is easy to consume 4,000 mg or more per day. Don't avoid sodium; just try to limit it. Replace salt with other spices to add flavor to your foods.

Total Carbohydrate

Fiber carbs are good for you, but other carbs will affect insulin levels and should be kept to less than ten grams per day. The higher the amount of sugar, the faster it will affect your blood sugar and insulin levels. The lower the amount of sugar, the slower the effects.

> *I have an easy rule of thumb that helps to determine the likelihood of releasing extra insulin: I take the total grams of carbohydrates on the food label, add the sugar grams, and minus the fiber grams. I call the result the insulin index. Between zero and ten is perfectly safe. If it is between ten and twenty, then it is possible you will release extra insulin. If it is between twenty and thirty, then it is probable and if it is over thirty, then insulin will definitely be released. Twenty is the magic limit to remember:*

Frequently Asked Questions and Myths

Q. I heard that if I stick to three colors on my plate that aren't white, cream, or yellow through such foods as fruits and vegetables, I will eat better?

A. Absolutely. This one makes great common sense.

Q. I heard that if I eat smaller meals every three or four hours rather than three large meals, I will eat less and stay leaner?

A. That depends on the size of the meals and what is in them. My approach calls for live food and no non-fiber, starch carb snacks during the day and only one large meal, eaten at the end of the day. I think you are more likely to overeat if you plan multiple meals. The fewer complete meals that you have, the less insulin you risk releasing. And I find it is a lot easier to plan one large meal per day rather than three, four or five smaller meals. After you have passed the adaptation stage and have transformed from "carb burner" to a "fat burner," you should no longer have feelings of deep hunger during the day. Occasionally, enduring periods of low-level hunger are good for you. When you are just a little hungry, you have more energy. Also, since you know you will be eating a big meal later, it is much easier to ignore a little hunger.

Q. I heard that if I cut down on soda, juice, and high-calorie coffee drinks, which are full of empty calories, I will stay leaner. Is that true?

A. Empty liquid calories are the worst. They enter the blood stream faster, spike your insulin very quickly, and don't really fill you up. If you really want a glass of soda, put it into your plan, but I have nothing good to say about soda. I drink only a limited selection of liquids. Water is fine anytime. Black coffee in the morning (1 cup), protein shake after workouts, and a glass of red wine in the evening with an occasional cup of all-natural tea to fill in any gaps. I drink other things from time to time, but not as part of my regular health plan.

Q. Can this lifestyle cure cancer, diabetes, arthritis, or any other diseases?

A. The only thing that can cure you is your body and its inherent healing potential. If your body is allowed to function with the least amount of stressors placed upon it, then it will be better equipped to fight any illness. Following the principles in this book will help you achieve optimal health.

Q. If I replace vegetable oil or canola oil with olive oil, will my diet will be healthier?

A. Yes. Vegetable and canola oils are very high in omega-6 fats, which are the wrong type of fats to consume.

Q. I still get hungry during the day, so what can I do to make it through to the next meal?

A. Eat. *But*—and this is very important—if you are hungry during the day, eat only live foods and avoid all non-fiber carbohydrates. If you eat non-fiber carbs, they will only add to your hunger and sabotage your plan. I always make sure to have live-food snacks available, such as avocado, nuts, eggs, and bee pollen. Remember, having a little hunger is good and tends to make you more alert and more productive. Mild hunger will pass, and that is a sign that your body has started to burn fat again.

Q. I heard that if I keep a food diary, if only for a couple of days per week, I will have more success losing weight and keeping it off.

A. Most people don't seem to recall what they ate, so keeping a diary of what you eat every day will help you identify where the problems are. However, if you are following this style of eating, you don't need to keep a diary. It's up to you.

Q. Is it true that eating turkey will make you tired?

A. Turkey contains a protein called L-tryptophan, and it is true that L-tryptophan can cause drowsiness. However, you would have to eat large amounts of turkey on an empty stomach, with no other proteins, for the sedative effect to occur. It is much more likely that the drowsiness you feel after a turkey dinner is due the high quantity of non-fiber carbs and other foods that are usually eaten with it.

About the Author

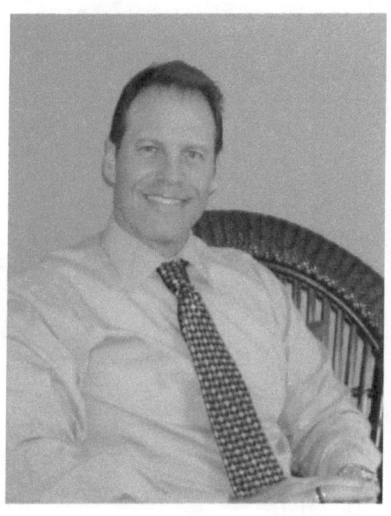

Dr. Bryan Craig is a natural-healthcare practitioner with an emphasis of Neuromyology and Nutrition, with over twenty years of experience. He has practiced in Florida, New York, and Arizona.

He earned his Doctor of Chiropractic from New York Chiropractic College in 1991.

In addition to his practice, Dr. Bryan Craig is a sought-after workshop presenter, guest lecturer, and writer.

Index

www.ingramcontent.com/pod-product-compliance
Lightning Source LLC
Chambersburg PA
CBHW031259280526
45784CB00004B/1911